ASYLUM OF THE GILDED PILL

THE STORY OF CRAGMOR SANATORIUM

Douglas R. McKay

Published by the State Historical Society of Colorado

© 1983 by the State Historical Society of Colorado. All rights reserved

Printed in the United States of America

ISBN 0-942576-26-8

SECOND PRINTING 1990

Library of Congress Catalog No. 83-61069

If a man were to tumble out of the heavens over Colorado Springs, he would drop into a natural health resort, and . . . he would derive some benefit from falling through the air.

Mountain Sunshine, 1899

CONTENTS

FOREWORD

When people talk about Colorado Springs and how it grew, they get rhapsodic about its founder General Palmer, the gold of Cripple Creek, Spencer Penrose, and the creature comforts of his Broadmoor Hotel. I am all for General Palmer and for gold and for Penrose, but this book of Douglas McKay's tells a far more exciting story—the neglected history of how Pikes Peak became famous and prosperous through its facilities for curing people of what ailed them. In particular, it tells how tuberculars found cures in the most charming ways at a place in the scrub oak north of town called Cragmor Sanatorium.

The renown of this institution from its opening in 1905 to its demise in the 1960s was due to the colorful physicians who ran it and to the just as colorful patients who found happiness and romance there as they cavorted their way back to health. Cragmor's founder was a tall, handsome, courtly Englishman, Dr. Samuel Edwin Solly, who made tuberculars feel better just looking at him. After Solly's death, Cragmor began its golden age under the direction of a young Virginian, Dr. Alexius M. Forster, who had managed TB sanatoriums far and wide. Dr. Forster believed that the best cure for TB was to take it easy, think beautiful thoughts, try a bit of romance—not too strenuous—and achieve "mental buoyancy" in the most elegant of possible environments.

Dr. Forster assembled a medical staff at Cragmor as glamorous as himself. It was headed by a handsome pioneer in developing TB antibiotics, Dr. Gerald Webb. Another staffer was a superb storyteller named Dr. Jack Sevier. Also present was a decorative lady-killer from Holland in charge of the sanatorium's lab work, Dr. Charles Boissevain.

Asylum of the Gilded Pill re-creates splendidly a passage in the history of Pikes Peak that may never happen again. But the lessons that Cragmor taught its patients survive in the minds of many residents of Colorado Springs today—how to appreciate the gift of life and how to enjoy it fully.

Marshall Sprague

PREFACE

Sixty years ago the Cragmor Sanatorium was a celebrated asylum for wealthy tuberculars. Many victims of the Great White Plague came from near and far to fill its handsome suites.

High on a field north of the Main Building was a large pithole intended for the disposal of medical paraphernalia—used sputum cups, empty bottles, soiled garments, and all of the discarded trappings of hospital convalescence. To that garbage heap one Saturday afternoon in the summer of 1924 stumbled two small boys from Papetown, joyously searching for treasures among the yucca and pines of Austins Bluffs. Discovering Cragmor's pile of trash, they were enthralled at the sight of several half-filled bottles of golden-yellow pills. Curiosity prompted them to take out and chew one or two of the enticing tablets, whereupon they found to their delight that the medicine tasted exactly like candy. They then proceeded to gobble up the remaining yellow pills.

One of the boys, complaining of stomach cramps, went home. Learning of his son's foolish encounter with the gilded pills, the father rushed the lad back to the sanatorium. He called for Dr. Forster, the resident director, demanding to know the content of the empty bottles. Forster reassured the anxious parent with words to this effect: "There's nothing to worry about. A stomach pump will not be necessary. Your son has swallowed nothing more than an excess of candy tablets." Explaining further, the doctor said, "These pills are a placebo. Their yellow coating merely gives the appearance of medicine. Since there's no known cure for tuberculosis, we often have to humor our patients a little. By swallowing these pills they believe they are getting well. As for your son, he likely has an old-fashioned bellyache from eating too much candy. A little rest, some fresh air and sunshine, and he'll be as healthy as most of our pill-popping patients."

That anecdote inspired the title for this book and is one of the many stories that kindled my research interest in the neglected but fascinating world of the Cragmor Sanatorium, the famous tuberculosis center of Colorado that flourished when "great expectorations" and euphoric dreams contributed in large measure to the human prosperity of Colorado Springs's amazing growth.

Asylum of the Gilded Pill is about the affluent, well-fed, generally sprightly health-seekers of Cragmor—their lust for fresh air, sunshine, gilded pills, and other fevered bodies. It represents the result of over one hundred firsthand interviews with former patients and employees of the sanatorium. It also reflects my reading of medical reports, admission records, memoirs, diaries, letters, news clippings, and institutional gossip columns. That which began as a casual search for a good yarn or two about regional medical practices and local folklore turned into a serious investigation of four years' duration, an effort to chronicle as reliably as possible Cragmor's inception, its preeminence among health resorts in the western United States, and its wretched decline amid clandestine abortions, undisclosed cases of syphilis, institutional mismanagement, and the humiliation of bankruptcy.

It should be understood that this narrative is a local history, based on documents assembled almost wholly from Colorado Springs sources. As such, it contains the hyperbole of early Colorado Springs boosterism. The reader is cautioned to weigh carefully the enthusiasm of my promotional sources (who exalted Cragmor as the best and the biggest, the first, and the most unusual) with the ironic reversal that reality so often accords to the mighty and strong, rendering the most unique, original, and influential palace a forgotten ruin on the sands of time, or leveling a once-inflated assessment of a distinguished individual to a present-day obsolescence. Indeed, there is much in this history to authenticate Percy Shelly's lines:

> Round the decay
> Of that colossal wreck, boundless and bare
> The lone and level sands stretch far away.

No effort was made to document thoroughly the medical history of Cragmor. I have avoided, for instance, any exploration into Dr. Gerald Webb's outstanding research and innovative developments both at Cragmor and at the Webb Tuberculosis Research Laboratory. I have also put aside Dr. Alexius Forster's impressive medical journals of a strictly professional character, concentrating instead on the more engaging human side of his lengthy directorship.

This account, then, attempts to recapture the authentic spirit of Colorado Springs's consumptive past, emphasizing the renown of Cragmor in the late twenties and early thirties and recounting the tragic deterioration and degradation of a once-celebrated resort. As such, I have relied more on oral histories than a stream of pedantic research reports and have taken special pains to corroborate my personal interviews. Also, my careful perusal of the intriguing private diaries and letters left by the major figures in the story has led me to focus more on the eccentricities of human behavior, sometimes perverse and always unpredictable, than to detail the solid, boring statistics of an institutional log.

A final word concerning the fortuitous preservation of some but not all of Cragmor's original records. Several years ago a rather arbitrary decision was made by the administration of the university campus that now occupies the site of the former sanatorium to destroy hundreds of valuable historical and genealogical records. As many old Cragmor files and records were being loaded on trucks destined for the city dump, I just happened to be walking by and inquired about the condemned materials. The campus custodians were only too happy to fill up my office with dozens of dusty tomes. And thus began a four-year research project of a most intriguing and rewarding kind.

Douglas R. McKay
Colorado Springs, 1982

NOTE TO THE SECOND EDITION:

Over the seven intervening years since this book was published, many of the fine elderly friends whose lives had touched mine in the course of researching Cragmor's past have passed away. Most poignant among those losses was Frieda Lochthowe, the Sanatorium's head nurse for many years and my most valued informant. It is to the memory of Frieda and other departed choice friends, without whom the fascinating history of the Cragmor Sanatorium could never have been written, that I affectionately dedicate this second edition.   DRM

ONE

Health Mecca of the West

*Colorado Springs is the best
resort on the face of the globe
for an invalid with lung disease.*
Louis R. Ehrich

Colorado Springs flourished on the bedrock of disease. While the gold mines of Cripple Creek helped to fill the coffers, pave the streets, and build the schools of General William Jackson Palmer's famous resort town, enduring prosperity came from its population of consumptives, the wheezing tuberculous invalids known as "lungers" or "chasers," who as health-seekers flocked to the city's hotels, tents, hospitals, and sanatoriums, grasping at the elusive vision of improved well-being.

They traveled from the metropolitan centers and country quarters of Canada, England, Germany, and Italy. They left the hospitals of New York, the rest homes of Boston, the boardinghouses of Baltimore, and the "Coughers' Flats" of Chicago. They came from every sector and recess of the eastern, southern, and midwestern United States, seeking miracle cures, absorbing the healing properties of Colorado's mineral springs and mountain sunshine, and responding to the fresh-air propaganda promoted by the region's pioneer physicians. Along with their diseased and wasted frames, they brought their families, their money, and their dreams. Many were so ill that they perished in a fierce rush of blood upon alighting from the train en route to their hospital beds. Others felt so frisky in the high mountain air, far removed from the distasteful life of smoke-filled rest homes back East, that they mounted horses, climbed to the top of Pikes Peak, fished, swam, and drank imported whiskey, then suddenly collapsed in a paroxysm of uncontrollable coughing or in the throes of a massive hemorrhage.[1] Yet many lived and prospered. With health restored and personal fortunes invested, they remained to build an incomparable pleasure resort along the eastern slope of the Rocky Mountains.

In the late 1950s a large banquet was held at the Antlers Plaza Hotel to honor many of the city's most distinguished longtime residents. The toastmaster invited the throng of opulent citizens to give an account of their reason for living in Colorado Springs. He asked all of those who had come to the region for their own health or that of some member of their family to raise their hands. Over 60 percent of the audience indicated that tuberculosis was directly or indirectly the reason for their residence in the city. Many had been mere children among the thousands of consumptive patients who some fifty years earlier had responded to a nationwide campaign to promote Colorado Springs as the most glorious health frontier in the world. Others had come in later years, when the largest and most celebrated sanatoriums were in their prime, each filled to capacity with tuberculous invalids. And for each person of prominence who had come to the city chasing the tonic cure, there were many more faceless, nameless individuals who came to cough and to bleed and to die. Those whose respiratory ailments were successfully treated generally remained as Colorado's adopted residents, while those who succumbed to the disease filled more than half of the plots at Evergreen Cemetery.[2]

Colorado Springs was known variably as the "TB Mecca of the West," "Sanatorium City," "City of Sunshine," "Sputum Hole of Humanity," or, less epithetically, the most delightsome place on earth in which to live—or die. Some of the city's most esteemed families can ascribe their move to Colorado to tuberculous bacilli: Bemis, Van Briggle, Glockner, Stone, Webb, Sprague—all were a part, at one time or another, of the consumptive procession. The largest stockholder in the world migrated to the city because of ill health, as did one of the country's most accomplished poets and novelists.[3]

Many wealthy tuberculars lived along North Nevada Avenue, known to the seven thousand residents of the city in the late 1880s as "Lungers' Row." These old homes still retain some backyard TB cottages. Elsewhere, especially on Wood, Tejon, and Cascade avenues, attached open-air porches can still be found, where afflicted members were isolated from the family to prevent contagion. The less affluent invalids of the convalescent society, among them hundreds of impecunious lungers without families or jobs, lived in crowded tent communities in or near the center of town. This fact prompted the unafflicted to fear contamination and hastened physicians to campaign vigorously for the establishment of remote countryside sanatoriums in which to house the indigent lungers.

The finest, best-equipped, heaviest-manned, and largest sanatoriums in the country were built on the outskirts of early Colorado Springs: Glockner (now Penrose Hospital) was established in 1890 and developed into the largest Catholic sanatorium in the country; Bellevue Sanatorium (now St. Francis Hospital) was begun in 1900, designed to be the world's largest Protestant tuberculous center; Nordrach Ranch (near the present site of National College), was founded in 1901 and enjoyed the distinction of being Colorado's first open-air sanatorium and the second such institution in the United States; Cragmor, today a campus of the University of Colorado, was officially opened in 1905 and thereafter became the most luxurious pleasure palace for well-to-do consumptives in the United States; Modern Woodmen of America, now the site of St. Francis Convent, received its first patients in 1909, the largest worldwide tuberculosis establishment conducted by a fraternal body; and finally, the Union Printer's Home, established by one of the nation's oldest national work organizations, eventually grew into the largest tuberculous care center operated by a labor society. There were at least ten other smaller sanatoriums nestled in the wooded back roads and the higher ranges of the Pikes Peak region. At one time the Colorado Springs area boasted the active operation of seventeen hospitals and sanatoriums.[4]

By the first decade of the twentieth century Colorado Springs was unique among communities in the world in terms of institutional and residential health care. If a stranger thought the city had no basic industries, he or she had only to calculate the enormous capital invested in sanatorium plants, the recreational institutions run by or for consumptives, the mineral baths, which attracted thousands of healthy tourists as well as diseased health-seekers, and the mountain drives, many constructed for the improvement of unhealthy lungs, to see that the industrial base of this community was as impressive as any other city of its size. Indeed, the health industry of Colorado Springs was as decisive, pervasive, and basic to its growth, character, and lasting prosperity as was the manufacture of steel to Pittsburgh, the making of flour to Minneapolis, or the distribution of goods to Kansas City.[5]

Owing to this steady migration of tuberculous health-seekers, Colorado Springs was blessed with the greatest crop of resourceful homesteaders ever assembled under the banner of disease. At times, however, the hacking migrants were a source of grave concern. Many newcomers to the Rocky Mountain boom town devoted themselves to social amusements, pursuing what Dr. Boswell P. Anderson called "wanton pleasure instead of health."[6] They were often looked upon as a scourge to public decency, as well as a threat to the public health of the community.

During its second decade of health-centered expansion, the city experienced such a severe housing shortage that prefabricated tent homes had to be shipped from Illinois. Masses of white canvas tents sprang up like early dawn mushrooms throughout the valley and in the mountain dales, giving rise to thriving resort towns, such as Green Mountain Falls, which was a veritable tent city in 1883. Other tent encampments were clustered unhygenetically in midtown parks, in the back yards of palatial homes, and along the rocky riverbed of Cheyenne Creek.[7] In response to this unsightly proliferation of tents, concerned citizens predicted a serious threat of contagion for the community, often backed by proclamations signed by physicians and public health officials. "If the swarming rate of the city's tent population increases," wrote one alarmed resident, "we will all perish in a horrible epidemic of tuberculosis."[8] Young schoolchildren mocked the tent dwellers at a downtown park, singing dreadful ditties about oral discharge and unseemly health practices. Those invalids who wantonly spewed sputum in close quarters were frequently victims of militant social excoriation. In one instance their tents were set on fire.[9]

Responding to the public hue and cry for improved sanitary regulations, in 1900 the editor of *Mountain Sunshine* declared,

"Large and more distinctive provisions must be made at once to accommodate the health-seekers who come in ever-increasing throngs."[10] It was this statement which, when read and mulled over by Dr. Samuel Edwin Solly, one of the city's leading health promoters, led to positive results. Then fifty-five years of age, Solly was considered second only to General William J. Palmer as Colorado Springs's most prominent citizen. An internationally recognized physician and without question the region's most successful public relations booster, owing to his published panegyrics on the merits of the Pikes Peak region as a health resort, Solly had long before determined to support any local movement or campaign that would redound to the city's financial and medical renown as well as to his own. The journalist's avid plea to build "larger and more distinctive provisions" merely rekindled an old fervor in Solly. He promised that the editor's entreaty would not fall on deaf ears. "I will personally see to it," he confided to the author of that 1900 petition, "that this beloved city, the very resort community to which I came in search of health twenty-six years ago, will be blessed by those provisions."[11]

That resolve gave rise to one of the most distinctive and peculiar health care institutions in the world: the Cragmor Sanatorium.

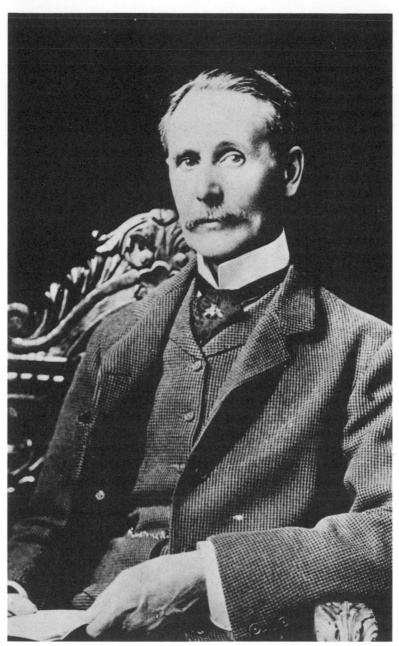

Dr. Samuel Edwin Solly

TWO

The Edwin Solly Era

> *Give me a hundred acres near*
> *town—a starter for buildings for*
> *a sanatorium, and I will guar-*
> *antee to make Colorado Springs*
> *the health resort of the world.*
> Samuel Edwin Solly

Edwin Solly had nurtured his elusive dream for a first-class sanatorium for many years. Indeed, this ambitious but basically conservative man silently coddled many idealistic aspirations, some of which fizzled for lack of time to nourish the creative spark, others for want of zeal to expand the flame. Occasionally his visions would burst into a glorious state of fruition. Whenever this intrepid dreamer persevered to promote his own name in the public's eye, he would know success. "Edwin Solly will never perish unheralded," reads a clipping found among his papers, "he believes too solidly in the virtues of his own mind."[1]

Such had been the case during Solly's seventeen-year tenure as president of the El Paso Club (1880–97), when he guided the expansion of a small and unpretentious fraternity into a grand organization of high social distinction, a club whose lavish balls, receptions, and exhibitions rivaled the most extravagant fêtes of Denver, New York, and Philadelphia.[2] Such too had been his experience between May of 1881 and June two years later, when that same goading urge for social prominence inspired Solly to devise the general plans of the celebrated Antlers Hotel,[3] and again in the late 1890s, when he promoted the founding of a first-rate golf course for Colorado Springs's prosperous citizens.[4] Solly was so intimately identified with the community in social affairs and public enterprises that he was often introduced and toasted as Colorado Springs's leading citizen. "Colorado Springs and Samuel Edwin Solly were inseparable in the late nineteenth century," wrote Billy M. Jones. "The town became world famous because the doctor, who had recovered his health there, gratefully and masterfully promoted it as a health resort for consumptives."[5]

Yet the aspiration that excited Solly's imagination above everything else had a long gestation period. It was a dream that took him over a quarter of a century to realize and at times it showed meager promise of fulfillment. In 1874, the year of his arrival from England, when his own physical stamina had been vitiated by tuberculosis and his first wife, Alma Helena, was on the brink of death with the same affliction, Solly first enunciated the desire that would absorb his professional interest for the rest of his days: the construction of a significant cure home for the treatment of tuberculosis. Displeased with the urban environment for health care in downtown Colorado Springs, where patients were often obliged to live in crowded boardinghouses or unsanitary tent colonies under the care of different doctors espousing different views on treatment, Solly hoped to establish a rural sanatorium complex, which would be located far from the dust and smoke of the city and run by a competent staff of resident physicians.

The dream was slow in coming. Eight plans were adopted, modified, and aborted during Edwin Solly's lifetime. Keen disappointment attended the rejection of each successive plan. No sooner did Solly endorse one proposal than costs would soar or support would dwindle, obliging him to await the adoption of yet another scheme.

The earliest attempt to establish a sumptuous sanatorium had been initiated as early as the spring of 1874. Under the auspices of the American Institute of Homeopathy, one of the oldest medical associations in America, an elaborate and highly ornamental edifice was designed, intended as a midtown hospital. It promised to be, as the *Colorado Springs Gazette* reported, "a great boon to those who come from abroad to gain their lost health in the invigorating climate for which Colorado, especially the Springs, is so justly noted the world over."[6]

This sanatorium was intended to be an ideal hospital in every way—spacious, innovative, and bold. It would command a prime location in the center of town, be three stories high, with deep frontage and exquisite landscaping, surmounted by a cupola, and surrounded on the front and sides by commodious porches and balconies.

Edwin Solly had just celebrated his twenty-ninth birthday when the announcement was made. Only a fortnight had passed since Colorado Springs's most recent health refugee had unpacked his luggage. As part of his welcome, Solly's medical colleagues invited him to express his professional views on certain features of the plan. He was understandably flattered, having been assured that he would have a personal role to play in the building's design.

Solly directed his attention to improving the open-air porch and cottage features of the proposal. He favored erecting corner sleeping porches and developing a series of small, home-like cottages to the rear of the building, arranged in a semi-circle, which was a concept that he had observed in operation several years earlier at Davos in the Swiss Alps. Solly had no way of knowing then that over the course of the next five decades that very concept of high-mountain TB treatment—the German fresh-air approach featuring outdoor porch areas for the tonic relief of respiratory ailments—would affect the entire architectural planning for public buildings and private homes throughout the Colorado Springs community.

Solly was committed to the philosophy that open-air convalescence represented the secret of success in the treatment of tuberculosis. It offered a twofold advantage, which was fully in consonance with his own outspoken views about high-altitude living. The first was to expose the invalid to the crisp and vital curative powers of the mountain air by sleeping in a well-ventilated, unheated room. "If fresh air is so important," went the popular saying, "then the more of it the better, even sleeping in tents at night, or canvas protected verandas, or in bedrooms with all the windows open."[7] The second advantage was that this provided patients and their families or attendants with comfortable quarters approximating the environment of home. From this European corner porch notion, which gave each lunger full access to fresh air, day and night, in any season of the year, Solly developed his own idea of a cluster of porches or screened cottages, each provided with the modest furnishings of a private home and designed to allow family members to reside with or near the stricken individual.

In his eagerness to popularize the idea that uninterrupted fresh air and sunshine, combined with the region's ideal altitude, were "nature's fortress built for herself against infection,"[8] Solly tended to disregard and at times oppose any kind of rest regimen. At one time he even espoused the idea of discarding physical rest altogether, stressing the need for tuberculous patients to exercise freely, to breathe deeply of Colorado's dry, cool, rarefied air, to sleep with their windows open, preferably on screened-in, unheated porches, and then to seek the solitude of an open-air cottage at a curative retreat or alone in the woods. One of Solly's successors at Cragmor, Gerald Webb, would come to regard such views as archaic, restrictive, old-fashioned, and downright dangerous, opposed to the value of strict bed rest. Nevertheless, there is no doubt that for some fifty years Edwin Solly's fresh-air prescription and stress on physical activity swayed the thinking of many physicians. Eastern doctors sent their patients to Colorado Springs on the strength of Solly's word alone. His influence was so pervasive, his reputation as an acknowledged authority on climate and its effects on diseased lungs so widespread, that his opinions, theories, and practices were heralded in every leading medical journal throughout the country and in Europe.[9]

Despite Solly's avid agitation for its construction, the midtown sanatorium project was abandoned. Numerous construction delays and rising costs unseated the plan. However, that disappointment failed to deter Solly in his eagerness to promote the porch and cottage concept throughout the city. He first set about constructing his own private cabin in keeping with that notion, locating the modest, wood-framed house on an elevated ridge some three hundred feet above the city at a site four and one-half miles from the center of town. That screened-in cabin, structured to expose the sleeping area to fresh air and sunshine, became the model for later fresh-air enthusiasts who developed small cottage colonies for consumptives in nearby mountain resorts. Solly coined a name for his summer retreat north of town: "the Cragmoor," a kind of nostalgic reminiscence of England, where the rocky bluffs and the open plain came together.

Solly frequently took his family and friends to the cabin. Friends and visitors from abroad found themselves obliged to admire the splendid view of the mountains and plain from atop the bluff above the retreat. And Solly himself repaired there alone for quiet weekend meditation and to read medical reports, write letters, and update his records. In later years he claimed that the great dream of his medical career gained impetus in that cabin. In May of 1879, while reflecting on the improvement that his countryside weekends had brought to his own diseased lungs, he considered "the benefits, both personal and professional, which other consumptives could derive from the erection of a chain of cottages, all comprising a health facility patterned after the German plan of open air sanatoria," snuggled among the craggy knolls of Austins Bluffs Park. There the disease could properly be treated. He wrote of that decision: "Attributing my own recovery from a long-term asthmatic condition and consumptive fever to the clean air, pure water and high altitude of the Cragmoor, I hoped to accord other tuberculous patients the same privilege."[10]

Solly pondered and shared that dream for more than twenty years. He spoke of it quietly among his medical colleagues. It filtered into his letters. It even became a favorite after-dinner subject with fellow trustees of the El Paso Club. Yet the years crept by and the doctor's dream remained little more than a passing fancy, occasionally clothed in eloquence. The demands of a heavy practice weighed on his time and sapped his energy. These included consulting commitments at St. Francis Hospital, the directorship of Bellevue Sanatorium, executive duties at the El Paso Club, numerous writing efforts, lectures to professional groups as near as Greeley, Colorado, and as far away as New York City, and the responsibilities pressed on him as president of four major medical societies.[11] Simply stated, there was no time to pamper his pet dream and thus the famous tubercular retreat he so fondly mentioned to his patients, friends, colleagues, and family was relegated to the domain of wishful thinking.

As the nineteenth century closed, Edwin Solly's sanatorium still remained unbuilt. He was now fifty-five. His assets, while substantial for a physician of the time, were not equal to the cost of constructing and equipping even a modest clinic, let alone a palatial hospital. And on top of everything else, Solly was beginning to show perceptible signs of a decreasing heartiness.

He spent a good part of the next two years (1900–1901) cultivating favorable responses to his sanatorium project. He discussed its details both privately and in public with established magnates of the gold rush era, with millionaire philanthropists, and with most of Colorado Springs's affluent citizens. The surprising fact is that in all these years of planning, designing, scheming, and dreaming, Solly never asked anyone directly for land or money.[12] If the natural reserve and polish of his English background could not permit such an abuse of etiquette, neither could his pride. Finally, though, at the insistence of his wife and armed with all of the convincing medical truths he had enunciated in several pamphlets on climatology, Edwin Solly decided to approach the man at the top—the founder and chief architect of Colorado Springs, General William J. Palmer.[13]

Palmer and Solly had been close friends from the time of Solly's earliest months of residence in the city. The young, ailing doctor had lost no time befriending and impressing his adopted city's founder. Solly's first publication praised the virtues of the region's mineral waters. Today that simple tract would be labeled opportunistic promotional literature, but in its time the publication, which pronounced the waters and climate of Manitou Springs salubrious in every respect, was recognized as a major contribution to medical knowledge. In its few pages Solly developed a persuasive thesis that the region offered healing powers that were unparalleled anywhere else in the world, its elevated climate was ideal for the treatment of respiratory diseases, and the salutary effects of bathing in and drinking from the area's soda springs were unequalled for physical and mental well-being. The section that especially delighted Palmer was Solly's rhapsodic endorsement of the local hotels, nature trails, trout streams, and amusement parks. With good reason Solly became Palmer's most trusted public relations man, and with equally good reason Solly could have turned to Palmer for financial support at any time. The surprising thing is that he had not seized an occasion to do so before.[14]

One afternoon in the fall of 1901 that belated occasion arrived. Solly and Palmer rode out to the Cragmoor retreat. They picnicked together outside Solly's cabin at the foot of a high ridge on the southwestern slope of Austins Bluffs Park—land that belonged by deed to General Palmer. Then they walked to

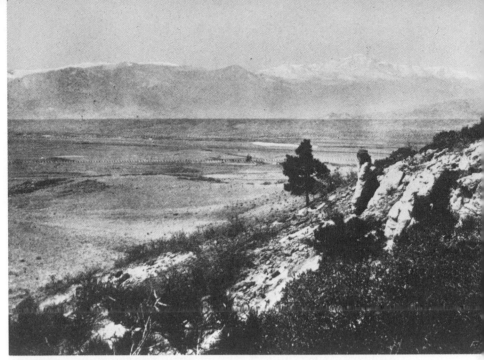

View from the future Cragmor site

the summit of a craggy knoll to admire the view of Pikes Peak as it loomed majestically above the pines and shrubs and prairie grass of the foothills below. Behind them stretched the undeveloped sheltered dale of the Garden Ranch, where vegetables would continue to be produced for another twenty years to satisfy the culinary needs of the Broadmoor. Before them, protected on the north and northwest by gradients of unrivaled beauty, the wide plateau that Solly had named "Cragmoor" sloped down to join the open red sand and the purple grass and brown scrub oak on the prairie below.

Solly spoke at length about his plan, stressing the necessity of mental quiet and poise in a country setting. He found, however, that General Palmer was no stranger to these ideas. During the past few weeks Palmer had been negotiating an important land transaction to donate ten thousand acres of Austins Bluffs Park to the citizens of Colorado Springs,[15] and enable one of Solly's medical colleagues, Dr. John White, to lease the William Otis home specifically for the establishment of a tubercular sanatorium. The Otis manor was located on the other side of the bluff.

Solly was unnerved by these tidings. In all of his discussions and deliberations about the need to build tubercular care centers, he had never imagined that someone else would actually outmaneuver him with a similar plan. And at this very time and next door to his own preferred site! Certainly others had broached the subject as energetically as he, urging the construction of consumptive hospitals. Dr. Samuel Fisk, dean of the medical school in Denver, had written lengthy monographs on the issue; Dr. Henry Sewell, an enthusiastic supporter of local sanatorium care, who only twelve years earlier had migrated to Colorado after working with the renowned Dr. Edward Trudeau at Saranac Lake, delivered frequent lectures on the need to build more stately consumptive mansions. Rabbi Friedman's marvelous Denver institution, the first free, nonsectarian hospital in the world for tuberculous invalids, was the recognized model for others to emulate throughout the region. Even Solly's close friend, Dr. Louis R. Ehrich, had been proclaiming for well over fifteen years that the one thing Colorado Springs most urgently needed was "a large, thoroughly equipped and commodiously arranged sanatorium."[16] The entire medical community concurred. Palmer's own personal physician, the genial and colorful Charles Fox Gardiner, was an outspoken advocate for the cause.

Yet it was neither the impulsive Gardiner, the outspoken Ehrich, the eloquent Sewell, nor the eminent Fisk who had turned Palmer's ear. It was none other than a quiet and unobtrusive country physician, Dr. John E. White, Solly's close friend and colleague, who not only was engaged in the same time-honored business of promoting a worthy idea, but who was about to assume command of a true-to-life rural sanatorium, not three miles away from Solly's cabin.

White wanted to establish a large tent settlement and bring sick lungers out of the city, giving them room to chase the cure far from indignant landlords and insensitive townsfolk. He would lease the William A. Otis estate, a palatial sixteen-room manor that adjoined the park's south front, to serve as the central building of his operation.[17]

This surprise disclosure prompted Solly to unleash an earnest plea for funds to support his own program, the first time in twenty years, he says in his private writings, that he had asked for money to launch his pet project. He explained that his sanatorium would not be operated as a tent community but would function as a closed sanatorium, a cottage colony, with a full resident staff of capable physicians. It would admit only curable patients who suffered from pulmonary tuberculosis and would put them on the road to a sure and rapid recovery in the dry and sunny air.

General Palmer was silent for several minutes. Solly later recorded that Palmer finally asked, "Tell me, my friend, just how much land and money will you need to build your sanatorium?"[18]

Palmer postponed announcing his gift and the location of Solly's preferred site for the sanatorium until mid-January of 1902. This allowed time to draw up the legal papers and form a board of medical advisors from around the country to enhance the public relations aspect of the sanatorium's early appeal.[19] Palmer entrusted the first formal news release about the transaction to his old friend, Samuel Francis, editor of the popular Colorado Springs magazine *Facts*. Francis promptly ran the following item on the third page of his January issue:

> General William J. Palmer has just given another evidence of his public spirit and generosity and of his abiding faith in Colorado Springs as a resort for health-seekers by offering 100 acres of land for a site for a sanatorium. In addition thereto he has offered the sum of $50,000 toward the $200,000 which will be necessary to build and equip the structure. General Palmer realizes, as many others do, that the real foundation for the enduring fame and prosperity of Colorado Springs is its splendid climate and the consequent attraction which it offers to invalids the world over. Conditions are found in this city which do not exist in any other resort in the known world. The high and dry site of the city, its magnificent scenic attractions, its sunshine and pure atmosphere, its social advantages, all combine to make the city singularly attractive to health-seekers.[20]

Nine days following the formal announcement of the grant, the Colorado Springs City Council recognized another generous donation by General Palmer, namely, his gift of ten thousand acres on Austins Bluffs Park designated for public recreational use, the same wooded retreat for picnickers and equestrians known today as Palmer Park.

That month of January 1902 was a time of unparalleled ebullience over tuberculosis in Colorado Springs. Consumption seemed more like a touristic commodity than a disease. Indeed, in examining the news reports, advertisements, and chamber of commerce propaganda of the time, it becomes increasingly apparent that tubercle bacillus was the city's major source of interest and income. New sanatoriums were extolled as a boon to the local economy and one physician joyously predicted that fresh waves of prosperous invalids would soon migrate to the area from the eastern seaboard. Several full-page spreads praised the pure air, outdoor tent life, and gracious living of Nordrach Ranch, with an accompanying plea to all so-called pukers to depart the warm, closed rooms of hotels and boardinghouses, forsaking "society with its attendant evils" in exchange for the salubrious atmosphere of forced feeding and prescribed exercise in the open air at Dr. White's country estate.[21]

Understandably, the influx of tuberculous hordes to the region also gave rise to occasional expressions of measured alarm. Dr. R. K. Hutchings, Solly's close associate and supporter, delivered a paper at the annual meeting of the Colorado Springs Chamber of Commerce on Friday, January 17, 1902, in which he proclaimed tuberculosis to be "beyond any doubt the greatest scourge of humanity," saying that "one person in every eight is afflicted at some stage of his life with one form or another of the disease, and dies of it." Hutchings then praised the city's absorbent sandy soil, its dry and sterile air, and the abundance of sunshine, all the while speaking reverently of Solly and his sanatorium plan. He concluded with a scathing invective against wanton spitters: "The health department has passed rules and regulations prohibiting promiscuous expectoration in any public place, or on the sidewalks. . . . Promiscuous expectoration is really the only source of danger . . . because the spit dries and is carried about in the air and the germ is breathed in. . . ." Hutchings insisted that all consumptives henceforth be required to use sanitary cuspidores or cheesecloth handkerchiefs, the same to be burned when soiled. To members of the Colorado Springs Chamber of Commerce, Hutchings was persuasive. Within a fortnight brick tablets inscribed No Spitting were issued as cornerstones for every new downtown edifice.[22]

The medical quacks too sought a piece of the new year's action. One of Solly's chief detractors was a boisterous medicine man named Francis Philips, who sold a sure-cure serum from his home-office at 24 North Tejon. Philips was one of Colorado Springs's most energetic ointment-rubbers, serum-shooters, and science-scoffers. He chose the same month of the announcement of Solly's new sanatorium to enlarge his own campaign of scorn against "all the heathen climate worshippers," while exalting with equal fervor the powers of his home-brewed product, the wondrous "Philips' Serum." Philips marketed his potion as "a new and certain cure for consumption": "It consists," he claimed, "of the inhalation of medicated vapors and the injection of Philips' Serum, tested and proven to cure from 70 to 90% of all cases of Consumption." Philips claimed it was simply suicide to depend on climate alone. Just call on him, pay for his treatment, and await the miraculous cure.[23]

The tubercle bacillus inspired local bards to praise the clean air and pure light of Colorado Springs. Ernest Whitney, the community's self-appointed poet laureate from Yale, published the following rhapsodic "Ode to Colorado Springs" in the Sunday *Gazette-Telegraph:*

> City of Sunshine! in whose gates of light
> Celestial airs and essences abound;
> City of Refuge! from whose sacred height
> Disease falls thwarted as a baffled hound,
> Loosing its fang, long burning in the wound;
> City of Life! thou hast a gift of years
> For all; swift Death a thousand times discrowned
> Within thy walls, and Fate, with waiting shears,
> Heed thee, as thou alone of earth didst feed their fears.[24]

The same editor who permitted Whitney's verses to grace the pages of the local press wrote an impassioned plea for invalids with limited means to stay out of Colorado Springs. He not only judged them to be a menace to health, but considered all indigent consumptives an aberration in the normal development of the community's prosperity. If woebegone consumptives could not afford Nordrach's rates or failed to pay the city council's imposed fines for promiscuous expectoration or found that their resources would not even defray the cost of Philips's guaranteed serum, they were summarily advised to stay out of the Pikes Peak region. The "City of Sunshine, Refuge, and Light" embraced with open arms the well-to-do health-seeker, but the penniless consumptive was as unwelcome as fool's gold in a Cripple Creek mine.[25]

What excitement abounded over this dreaded killer of statesmen, princes, and poets! Bacteria was the talk of the town. A sanatorium explosion was under way in 1902. Medical organizations met frequently to discuss plans to build large, splendid hospitals. The chamber of commerce devised clever publicity schemes to lure monied invalids to the area. The city council appropriated liberal allowances for the maintenance of the municipal health department. At every turn fortunes were squandered—or invested—to publicize Colorado Springs internationally as a magical mecca for the restoration of broken health and ailing lungs. Even physicians were commissioned and paid large sums of money to write telling truths about the region's energizing climate, its incomparable air, and the healing properties of its waters. In March the city spent $3,500 to purchase a seventeen-ton steamroller, which was the largest single expenditure that the council had approved in years. And for what reason? Because the community's leading doctors insisted that the dust on the downtown streets was so pernicious to troubled lungs that it had to be settled at once by moisture and a mechanical press. Indeed, no expense was too great, no effort too taxing, to build and maintain the image of the Springs as an incomparable haven for affluent tuberculars.

Edwin Solly's thoughts paralleled this surge of public interest to entice wealthy invalids to the region. When asked late in February how his construction plans were progressing, he replied, "We will build the sanatorium on the large scale planned." Soon afterwards he announced that the name "Cragmoor" had been officially approved, and would henceforth grace all maps of the area.[26] He then solicited and was granted positive editorial endorsements for the project from the local press.[27] Finally, he initiated a vigorous campaign to raise money "for the eventual expenditure of not less than $350,000."[28]

Solly took his first appeal for funds to the El Paso County Medical Society where, as president, he delivered a forceful address on the objectives of the proposed sanatorium. That pronouncement in March was followed by the distribution of thousands of printed copies of the report, which were mailed to local and out-of-state physicians and to prospective patients throughout the world.[29]

Solly's bold monetary plea, designed to solicit subscriptions of large amounts "to aid the philanthropic plan," started out in high gear. His main argument to would-be supporters at home was that "the new sanatorium would advance the prosperity of the city and its inhabitants." He assured the community that once the new patients moved into the area, many would remain permanently, "brought into Colorado as citizens through the gateway of the sanatorium." The language he employed to appeal for money took an eloquent turn: "There may never be any material benefit to the one who subscribes, but he will ever have the satisfaction of knowing that he has conferred a boon on humanity and perhaps taken the canker of fear and dread from some poor heart and placed therein instead a white rose of hope." To those from the midwestern and eastern states and Europe, principally the individuals he hoped would comprise the better part of Cragmor's prosperous population, Solly directed requests for substantial financial support. "Patients who are able should pay handsomely for what they receive," he said.

The 1902 report also provided clear hints of Solly's intention to build the biggest and best sanatorium in the world. He spoke of "varied and accessible open air accommodations, spacious grounds, extensive graded walks with resting places," but his primary concern was to establish a health citadel without par: luxurious, stately, and high-priced. He wrote that "while the cost of maintenance will be higher, the rates charged can also be higher, probably averaging $30 to $35 a week."[30]

One skeptical colleague, the distinguished Dr. William H. Bergtold of Denver, took Solly to task for his elitist views. Standing before the assemblage at the El Paso County Medical Society, Bergtold exclaimed that it would make better sense to build places for the poor rather than for the rich. He argued that Solly's sanatorium, intended only for the wealthy, would deny health care to the poor, to which Solly replied, "The only way to keep a sanatorium for the poor running successfully is first to establish one for the rich and make it foot the bills for its less fortunate brother."[31]

To these words followed shouts of "Hear! Hear!" from the audience. Bergtold continued to argue for an institution capable of serving the indigent but he was clearly outnumbered. Most of Colorado Springs's affluent citizens and influential physicians rallied behind Solly, among them James A. Hart and Will Howard Swan, both of whom spoke earnestly in support of the palatial plan "to give this city the prominence it deserves." The medical society then voted overwhelmingly to endorse Solly's proposal, choosing to build first for the wealthy, then from the profits subsidize a later edifice designed for the poor. Bergtold, obliged to rest his case, had to wait nine years before his view found a responsive ear in the Springs, and only then because social discord forced the issue into public debate.

Having secured local support—or at least assent—Solly endeavored at once to commission the most versatile, respected, and expensive architect in town to design a mansion worthy of his thirty-year vision. For this task he engaged the unflappable Irishman Thomas MacLaren. Since his migration to Colorado nine years earlier due to ill health, MacLaren had established himself as the community's foremost architect.[32] He was receptive to all of Solly's suggestions and particularly intrigued by the doctor's energetic insistence that sleeping porches be the focal concern of the bedroom units. Modeled after the same plan that Solly had worked out in blueprint form many years before, when the midtown sanatorium was first proposed, MacLaren designed a structure teeming with open-air porches of generous dimensions.[33] Solly so harangued his architect about sunlight and fresh air that MacLaren himself became a disciple of the sun philosophy. Many of his future constructions in Colorado Springs, as well as his designs for sanatoriums outside of town, Sunnyrest and Modern Woodmen of America, would reflect the Solly view of mountain living.

For Solly's inimitable Sun Palace at Cragmor, MacLaren was charged with the task of situating all of the rooms for invalids on those sides of the building that faced the sun. Likewise, the dining rooms, designed to occupy the whole of the first and second floors of the southeast wing, were so arranged that three sides could be thrown open to the outside. The mammoth entertainment hall, which filled two floors of the southwest wing, was designed to serve the same function. Dotted about the grounds were shelters, arbors, and benches so that, as Solly explained, "patients would be encouraged in every way to lead, by day and by night, an outdoor life."[34]

As for the main building, it was in general U-shaped, with wings projecting at a sixty-degree angle to equalize sunlight exposure time to the rooms and form an effective shelter from easterly or westerly winds. An attractive garden faced the south, which was enclosed by three sides of the edifice. Entry to the building was on the north side beneath an elegant porte cochère. Public reception rooms, a lounge, a billiard room, the library, and the amusement hall and dining room complex occupied the first floor. Projecting off the main building toward the north were the kitchen units, which were isolated from the other areas of the sanatorium.

Solly made no effort to hide his resolve to build the foremost health resort in the world. Preliminary figures placed the estimated cost of the building between $300,000 and $350,000, a soaring amount for construction in that era. Yet by the time MacLaren completed his plans, the higher estimate had nearly doubled. According to Solly, no construction could begin until the Cragmor association had at least $100,000 on hand; however, after four months of aggressive campaigning, only $12,000 above the base sum of $50,000 first donated by Palmer had been raised. Solly had solid verbal pledges but the actual financial support had yet to appear.

Solly was abashed. He had no recourse but to delay construction. In reality, the scheme was too grandiose, too overcharged with quixotic fervor, too embellished with Edwin Solly's unquenchable need to build the stateliest cure center on the globe. It was simply too vast a venture to warrant subsidy by philanthropic means. The local citizenry protested that Cragmor's fees would limit admission to all but the most affluent consumptive tycoons, while most of those tycoons, whoever they were, still seemed to prefer the rich cream, exotic yodel, and crisp alpine air of a Swiss chalet near Davos to the uncertain magic of Colorado's tuberculosis haven.

However, despite these setbacks, Solly kept chasing after his dream and raising money. On February 26, 1903, he submitted his completed plans for the Cragmor Sanatorium to a committee representing the Real Estate Exchange, the Merchants' Association, the Mining Exchange, and the El Paso Medical Society.[35]

To allay the growing concern among the committee members, many of whom had pledged considerable money for Solly's Sun Palace, over construction delays, unconfirmed expenditures, rumors about recent changes in design, and conflicting reports on the current status of Solly's fund-raising drive, Solly was pleased to inform them that $80,000 had been subscribed for the project, MacLaren had modified downward the cost estimate on the main building, and work would soon commence on the construction of satellite cottages to be used to receive patients while awaiting the erection of the Sun Palace.

Some of the businessmen voiced apprehension that the continuing lack of a single large sanatorium in the city was creating an unwelcome burden on the facilities of the Glockner Sanatorium. Glockner was a popular care center that combined many hospital features with an overcrowded tubercular ward and twenty-seven convalescent tents on its western slope. It was then adding new wings, including a spectacular sun parlor that resembled a large greenhouse, designed to accommodate the many TB patients demanding medical service.[36] Others on the committee were troubled by alleged reports that Nordrach Ranch imprisoned terminal patients in the most wretched tents ever devised for human torture and were concerned that Solly treat his patients more humanely than done at Nordrach. Solly countered that he agreed fully with Dr. White's open-air methods: "I practice them myself," he wrote, in answer to the frequent criticism that subzero temperatures did nothing to arrest consumption but only froze the victims of the disease to death.[37]

Solly's decisive manner waylaid much hostility, calmed a few anxieties, and replaced mounting distrust with new assurances. Nevertheless, the overriding concern at the newly formed businessmen's association, organized as "a community advisory board for local sanatoria construction," was the town's burgeoning population of wheezers. Solly had to address the crucial problem of overcrowded facilities. Until Cragmor was operative, even provisionally, the city faced an alarming deficiency of adequate health care.[38]

Already Colorado Springs's inhabitants numbered 35,500. Sick people were pouring in by the droves, seeking immediate lodging, demanding medical attention, and creating serious health hazards in their improvised tent dwellings downtown. Of

greater concern to the politicians was the fact that increasingly
the city was coming under national scrutiny; famous people
from the East visited the region every month of the year. Within
ten days of that February 26 business meeting, the intrepid fem-
inist Carrie A. Nation would be in town. And in early May—
just five weeks ahead—the great Theodore Roosevelt with his
entourage of holiday sportsmen would sweep into the most famous health and pleasure resort in the Rockies. Solly felt pressure from all sides—the business world, concerned citizens,
fellow colleagues, and municipal government. His project, despite inordinate high costs, had to go forward. The committee
agreed that the Cragmor Sanatorium was needed to alleviate
a desperate social and medical need. Solly was petitioned,
therefore, to be more precise about the work. Time was of the
essence and the businessmen demanded more specific information. Consequently, before the meeting adjourned the doctor requested one week's time in which to confer with his architect;
he would then return to file a definite construction plan before
the joint session of the association.

True to his word, Solly returned to face the restless citizen
council the following Saturday evening, March 7, 1903. "The
work will be pushed with such vigor that within a year's time
patients will be received by Cragmor," he confidently an-

Dr. Solly in his downtown residence-office

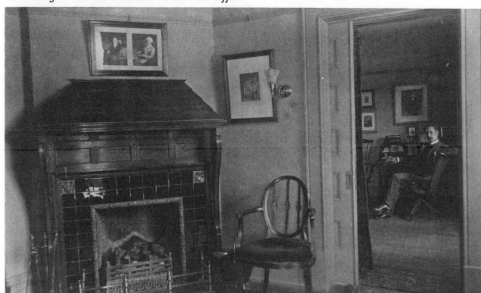

nounced. "The general plans for the Main Building and in fact for the entire structure have been completed and accepted, and it is our intention to build the central block as soon as Architect MacLaren can draw the specific plans, so that contracts may be let. All of this should be effected within five months."[39]

Someone then asked Solly what the adjusted cost would be for the Sun Palace. His response: "It will cost about $100,000. In time, as we raise more money, we will add wings to the new edifice."[40] Solly and MacLaren had thus found the answer to their plight over time and financial constraints. They would build only as much as the available funds could pay for, then await a fresh flow of charitable donations to complete the full scheme.

The doctor reminded his anxious constituents that no stock would be sold but funds for the erection of the sanatorium would be raised by voluntary contributions. Perhaps to satisfy the contingent that still opted for a poor people's nonelitist hospital, Solly reiterated that his plan was "to use the profits derived from running Cragmor to erect and maintain a similar institution for the poor."[41] However sincere that intention may have been, it was never carried out, neither in Solly's lifetime nor thereafter.

During the week between Solly's two formal appearances before his critics, MacLaren had made significant reductions in the size of the modified Sun Palace. He consolidated the enormous dining rooms into one space, converted the opulent entertainment hall into a modest assembly room, and diminished the recreation area—the library, billiard room, and lounge—into a single large room that he called the "covered porch." This porch would overlook sunken gardens occupying a space 200 x 150 feet, open out over a terrace to the south, and be enclosed by two cloisters. The smaller building, however, still retained its original regal image. And notwithstanding curtailed dimensions everywhere, MacLaren managed to increase, at Solly's behest, the floor space of each patient's suite by twenty-eight square feet.

Throughout the ensuing months, while construction bids were slowly coming in, Solly busied himself with local public relations activities and visits to the East Coast to woo converts to his promised land. "Cragmor truly possesses Edwin," his wife observed. "It is constantly on his mind. He fills his suitcase with brochures instead of clothes. Through the Midwest, up and down the East Coast, it is nothing but Cragmor, Cragmor, Cragmor."[42]

Meanwhile, urban quacks back home were promoting such a rash of tantalizing cures for consumption as to incense the community's responsible physicians. Upon returning to Colorado Springs Solly joined his colleagues in a staunch battle to educate the diseased population concerning the evils of the rampant brews, nocturnal injections, perfumed inhalations, and syrupy serums. One such marvel, a home treatment tagged "Antidotum Tuberculose" but known popularly as the Bensonizer Cure for Tuberculosis, which was promoted by hundreds of impassioned testimonials printed in local newspapers, invaded Colorado Springs about this time from Kalamazoo, Michigan. This wonder treatment, so claimed one full-page advertisement, "has changed invalids from shadows of manhood to strong men, from mere wisps of women into plump, full-chested maidens and matrons, the new lease of life for the thin, pale, hopeless sufferers in the very shadow of the Tomb. If you have that horrible heritage, a death taint in the blood . . . write! It is your sacred duty to stop the encroachment of this terrible disease before it is too late."

Another popular cure-all was Duffy's Pure Malt Whiskey, highly prized by the area's boozing consumptives. "Death is Near!" ran the typical headline banner announcing this miracle drink. "Such cases are happening every day, and every one of them can easily be cured by Duffy's Pure Malt Whiskey. It cures coughs, colds, consumption, grip, bronchitis, and pneumonia. . . . It prolongs life, keeps the old young and the young strong. . . . This is a guarantee. $1.00 a bottle, one teaspoonful in a half glass of water every two hours."[43]

Solly delivered a series of widely publicized addresses to counter the effectiveness of local charlantry. He rebuked the false promises with the vengeance of an aroused Hippocrates. "Nowhere is the invalid fool more surely or promptly punished for his folly than in Colorado," Solly remarked.[44] To warn consumptives against local quackery, Solly was fond of telling the story of a young Jewish boy, a recent patient of his. The lad had arrived in Colorado Springs a few years before, badly frightened. He had not yet finished his trade and had little money to maintain himself. Impatient with the prolonged rest that seemingly failed to bring relief, the boy "fell into the hands of some medical fakirs, who rapidly seized his little cache of money." His nervous tensions increased, his disease worsened, and he died.[45]

Another of the doctor's favorite exemplary tales concerned a young man of twenty-two who came to Colorado from the East. The year before he had been made a partner in his father's business, and everything seemed fair for him when it was discovered that he had consumption. When he reached Colorado Springs he was dead drunk; he had been in that condition since he had heard the doctor's verdict. Though Dr. Solly straightened him out for a while, the fellow had no control. One evening he drank several bottles of local firewater, the kind guaranteed to cure tuberculosis, flung himself into several wild nights of adventures, and went home "cured." Solly then hammered home the fitting moral denouement: "The next summer the lad was readmitted, but he died on the way to the hospital with a massive hemorrhage."[46]

Battling the home-brewed witch doctors was only one of Solly's endeavors while waiting for the final bids on the Sun Palace. He was also concerned about the little attention given to hygiene in local dwellings and the unsatisfactory supervision of boardinghome sufferers, problems that presented new dangers of infection to the city's able-bodied inhabitants. Solly was especially worried that his eastern colleagues would dissuade their wealthy patients from visiting the region because the town was too full of sick people. He also showed a hard-line conservatism by launching an attack on "the social gayety of the town," which in his opinion "encouraged the invalids to lead too exciting and careless a life."[47]

Concerned as well with the extraordinary growth of the town, which in its thirty-third year boasted the presence of thirty-five millionaires and had the reputation of being one of the most aristocratic communities in the country, Solly saw this commercial prosperity as partially a bane to good public health. Growth and prosperity gave rise to greater use of the streets, causing the traffic to grind up the roadbed into dust; generated a large and ever-increasing amount of smoke, which interfered with the good progress of diseased lungs; and caused the proliferation of unsuitable boardinghouses and hotels. These factors, he felt, made eastern physicians warier about sending their patients to live in Colorado.

Emerging from Solly's social betterment campaign was a groundswell of community pressure on the city council, with requests to adopt sterner measures to abate the smoke and dust nuisance in the city. Automatic stokers were soon applied to large furnaces, while those who stoked smaller furnaces were instructed to put on the coal more frequently and in smaller quantities at a given time.[48]

Underlying his community involvement, of course, was Edwin Solly's untiring argument that the construction of Cragmor on the grand scale proposed would reduce health risks and improve community well-being. The colorful and influential Charles Fox Gardiner echoed Solly's theme. He too warned the population that unless Cragmor was built soon, the new resorts springing up in New Mexico and Arizona might outflank the city's fading reputation as the land of miracles. "We have competitors which seriously endanger our prosperity as a health resort," he would soon declare.[49] As usual, Edwin Solly could count on Gardiner's salty competitive spirit to persuade his townspeople in the best tradition—that old hometown prosperity gag. And it always seemed to work.

Nevertheless, the winter months of 1903 approached and still no building contract had been awarded. Costs had zoomed so high in consequence of the inflated price of materials and the disturbed state of the labor market that Solly considered the wisdom of postponing construction again until the outlook was more favorable. Moreover, sufficient money had not been subscribed to equip the central block adequately, that portion of MacLaren's more than seventy sheets of plans that Solly was especially eager to erect. As the new year came on, Solly realized that the cost of the Sun Palace would be prohibitive unless additional modifications were made. He reluctantly asked MacLaren to reduce its size by omitting the assembly hall and one-half of the dining room area. "At this rate," Solly lamented, "we will be left with nothing but a breeze sweeping through an empty frame."[50]

Eventually only the breeze remained. The cost of erecting the central building was so disproportionately high to Solly's envisioned plan that, in despair, he abandoned the notion of constructing his sumptuous Sun Palace, deferring instead to Thomas MacLaren's suggestion that several small pavilions be built in its place. The original plan had called for the arrangement of cottages radiating out from the main building in a wide crescent, each equipped with suites facing south, with Solly's beloved sleeping porch alongside and a private bathroom behind the porch. To that aspect of the project Solly finally had a firm building contract. He then assured his critics that his decision was the right one: "While the accommodations will be superior in comfort and pleasantness so as to suit the most fastidious, yet there will be no waste of space or money for mere ornamentation or display." Though disappointed that his Sun Palace would have to be shelved, perhaps indefinitely, Solly still insisted that "Cragmor unquestionably will be the best sanatorium in all aspects that so far has been built, containing everything needed for the most efficient treatment of tuberculosis."[51]

Construction began in the late spring of 1904. Then countless delays followed: labor disputes, foul weather, bad roads, ill health, inertia. The opening, first scheduled in October of that year, was postponed until January, then again until March, and finally until June.

The Cragmor Sanatorium formally opened its doors to its first consumptive patients on June 20, 1905. According to the most reliable report, the complex of pavilions, cabins, and auxiliary edifices represented an investment of $30,000, a far cry from the bloated figures that had accompanied the plan for a large central building.[52] Solly's original summer cabin—the rest home of his own consumptive past—was remodeled. Behind it on a level spot just under the steep rise of the bluff loomed the administration and recreation building. It contained a dining hall, parlor, kitchen, servant's quarters, and offices, with wide verandas on the south, east, and west, surrounded by lawns, flowers, trees, and shrubs. On either side, also aligning the bluff, stood twin frame pavilions, two stories high, each equipped with eight suites for tuberculous guests. Each of the sixteen units had its own private sleeping porch, which was positioned to allow direct sunlight and fresh air to flood the room behind. Eight single wooden frame cabins, similar in construction to Solly's retreat cottage of nearly thirty years before, were scattered about the hillside, each with one room and an adjoining sleeping porch. About the grounds were tree-lined shelters and stone or wooden benches and to the south MacLaren had designed an ample horse stable, a laundry house, and a two-story dormitory for outside help.

A description of the setting, warmly sketched by Solly himself, appeared in the New Year's Eve edition of the 1905 *Colorado Springs Gazette:*

> The Cragmor Estate consists of a park of 110 acres, 400 feet above the town. It is nestled in a cove upon the southern slopes of a bluff which runs east and west rising some 200 feet behind it. Thus it is sheltered from the north and northwest. The bluff is covered with crags, pines, shrubs and turf, the soil of the slopes and valley is sand and gravel; there is no water in the soil, the abundant and pure water supply being brought for fifteen miles in pipes from the mountains. This situation, owing to its greater height and distance from the mountains, makes a later sunset by half an hour than in the city. Behind and to the east of it is a broken country of bluffs and valleys stretching for miles to the divide towards the north and merging into the great plains to the east.
>
> A magnificient panorama of mountain and plains opens before it; the mountain view extends southward for a hundred miles. Gently sloping paths on the bluff behind lead upward to still more entrancing views.
>
> No habitations or dusty roads are near it and yet the busy town and hurrying trains are seen, while a station on the Atchison, Topeka and Santa Fe railroad is only a mile away, and the electric cars a further mile beyond.[53]

The first guests admitted among Cragmor's twenty-four inaugural consumptives were seven of Solly's private patients. The thrill of their long-awaited admittance was somewhat dampened, however, by the sad news that their beloved doctor was critically ill.

During the last phase of the sanatorium's construction period,

shortly before its opening, Solly fell prey to a chronic neuras-
thenic collapse, the result of general fatigue aggravated by the
trauma of his arduous work. While Cragmor had given Solly a
dramatic zest for life in his final years, the tensions he un-
derwent during its planning stage had undermined his health.
Sheer exhaustion confined him to bed through most of the fall
of 1905. While only sixty years of age, Solly presented the aspect of a very old man to those who stopped by to wish him
well. Thomas MacLaren hardly recognized his friend. In a later
letter to Elizabeth Solly, MacLaren referred to his last visit with
her husband: "It seemed as though Edwin had already died
with the completion of Cragmor. When that lifelong mission of
his was over, his tired old frame just withered away."[54]

At the insistence of his wife, as soon as Solly was sufficiently
strong to withstand the journey, the family departed for Florida
to spend the winter months of 1905. The brief rest seemed to be
so beneficial that Solly returned to Colorado in April of 1906
with renewed determination, though lacking the old vigor. His
stamina, however, had been severely weakened. He announced
the end of his medical practice, bid farewell to Cragmor, and
moved to Asheville, North Carolina, to be under the care of his
stepson, William H. Evans. There he languished, rallied for a
while, lapsed again, and eventually succumbed to complications
of age and pneumonia. At sixty-one years of age, on November 19, 1906, Samuel Edwin Solly died. His body was shipped
by train to Colorado Springs where it was met by his wife, two
daughters, two stepchildren, and a large delegation of close
friends and fellow colleagues from the El Paso Medical Association. Following a large public service at St. Stephen's Episcopal
Church, Solly was interred in a private service at Evergreen
Cemetery.[55]

One week after his death, the *Colorado Springs Gazette* hon-
ored Edwin Solly in one of the last public eulogies to carry his
name. "He was one of our institutions," the editor wrote. "It
was largely due to him that Colorado Springs has been for years
one of the best known of American cities. . . . It is owing to him
as much as to any other man that physicians in every part of
the United States know about Colorado Springs and its health-
giving qualities, beautiful surroundings, and excellent society. . . . Dr. Solly's most enduring monument will probably be

Cragmor Sanatorium. To that he had given of his best efforts. He had looked forward for years to the establishment of an institution of the kind, and it must have been a great gratification to him that it should be finished and in successful operation before he passed away."[56]

It is one of those curious ironies of local history that the city whose magic and beauty Solly had proclaimed to the world so soon forgot him. As the years passed and Cragmor became one of the country's foremost sanatoriums, the memory of Edwin Solly was quietly pushed aside. Other names replaced his as new leaders and developers of Cragmor came and departed: Gerald B. Webb, Alexius M. Forster, Otto Einstein, George T. Dwire. For a long time the original cottage he had built for himself on the bluff, twice remodeled and expanded before 1910, did carry his name—"The Solly." It was the only visible token of a community's remembrance of that gentle man, prominent citizen, clever opportunist, able promoter, and founder of a successful cure center for thousands of tuberculous patients. Today there is not a street, city park, public building, or historical plaque anywhere in the Pikes Peak region, with the modest exception of one painting in the El Paso Club, to extol the name or notable achievements of Samuel Edwin Solly, Colorado Springs's second son.

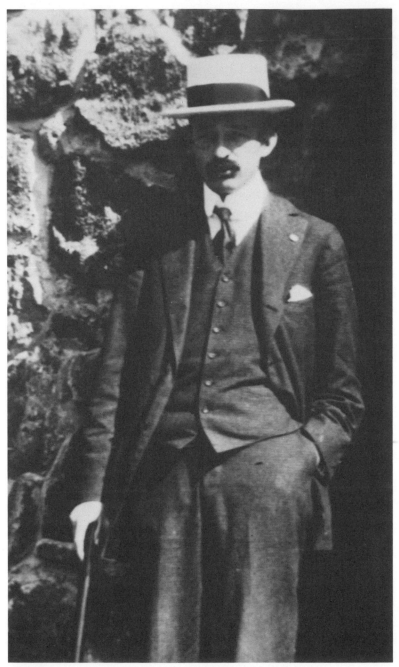

Alexius M. Forster, the dapper young doctor of Cragmor

THREE

The Days of Dr. Forster

The physician is the keystone
of the institution, and by him
our sanatorium stands or falls.
Laurence L. Cragin

Solly's illness and death were damaging to Cragmor's retarded opening. Indeed, the sanatorium suffered the shock of a still-born debut. While in July of 1905 every unit had been filled to capacity, by November of the following year—the month Solly died—the Cragmor cure house resembled a ghost town infirmary more than the distinctive monument its founder had visualized. Its population had shrunk from twenty-four handpicked invalids to ten tanned and testy fops, and even they were asked to leave. In one of Solly's last public statements he declared that "the physician in charge must have the power to dismiss a patient when the rules are not obeyed."[1] Left without a resident director, Cragmor rapidly deteriorated, thanks to a handful of vain and debauched dandies who broke all of the house rules and impeded the progress of the medical program.

However, the event that forced the callow institution to close its doors for eight months had little to do with Solly's departure or any subsequent mourning of his loss. More directly affecting the institution was an accident that occurred at the Garden of the Gods, a narrative known well by all who respond to accounts of heroism, namely, William J. Palmer's fateful fall, at age seventy, from the back of a squatty cow pony named Scrub Oak. The accident resulted in the irreparable severance of three cervical vertabrae, an almost total paralysis from the neck down, and the threat of imminent death.[2]

Dr. Will Howard Swan, who within one year's time would

become one of Cragmor's trio of new directors, was General Palmer's attending physician. Swan was responsible for concocting the marvelous India-rubber water bed that provided a measurable degree of comfort for Palmer during the early agonizing months when the old gentleman's life hung in the balance. Palmer, through his own great will power and aided by superior medical attention, survived for almost thirty months. Nevertheless, his accident engaged the full attention of the medical community, so much so that Cragmor's dreary isolation went unheeded. Front-page reporting reflected little concern for any problem beyond Palmer's condition as he hovered near death under the care of Will Swan, Henry C. Watt, and a team of medical consultants and nurses at Glen Eyrie Castle.

As for Cragmor, the institution was suddenly an orphan. Within one month it had lost both parent and godfather. There was no one to take charge. The medical advisory board of the Cragmor Sanatorium Association numbered fourteen physicians, but only one member of the board actually lived in Colorado Springs and his private practice allowed him no time as surrogate director. The semiattended asylum was run for a short time by Dr. P. A. Loomis, a youthful protégé whom Solly had hired to assist him during Cragmor's first tentative year of operation, aided by a very supportive but inexperienced woman named Miss M. C. McHaffey. Their patients were principally young men, only moderately ill, and wretchedly spoiled by the possession of too many material assets. Loomis had the additional burden of trying to begin his own medical practice in town. His administrative talent was clearly deficient; at one time he admitted four new patients without learning their names! Mail was left unanswered, the grounds were uncared for, and the laundry and meal service fell into chaotic mismanagement. With Palmer lying in dire straits at Glen Eyrie and the medical community's anxieties flooded with turmoil, no one stepped forward to assume the responsible command of Cragmor. Thus the new sanatorium closed its doors within a fortnight of its founder's demise, moribund in its infancy, subject to harsh winter storms and vandalism.[3]

Over the winter months of 1906–1907, Cragmor deteriorated rapidly. It seems incredible that such a newly built and promising establishment, the result of many years of sacrifice, planning, and labor, would be permitted to suffer the indignities that looting, damage, and neglect heaped upon it. In the early spring of 1907, when three members of Cragmor's board of trustees gathered at the deserted cottage colony to survey the grounds, they found the unattended buildings in a state of wretched disrepair: broken panes, ripped screens, stolen furnishings, vandalized equipment. One of the eight frame cabins had burned to the ground, due either to malicious mischief or a lightning assault.

J. Arthur Connell, an enterprising Scot from Edinburgh who had made his Colorado fortune in ranching and real estate and who was then president of Colorado Title and Trust Company (the organization holding the deed to the Cragmor property) insisted that immediate reparations be made and that the association hire a full-time watchman to forestall further abuse. Soon afterwards the trustees agreed to restaff Cragmor and admit a handful of carefully selected patients. By May new articles of incorporation were filed. Thereafter the premises buzzed again with activity: hammers pounding, mops swabbing, brushes slopping paint. Renovations were executed quickly and thoroughly. Several new hillside cabins and ten convalescent tents were added, increasing Cragmor's capacity to around thirty patients.

A mild-mannered easterner named J. J. Mahoney, whose most recent employment as director of the Massachusetts State Sanatorium for Tuberculosis at Rutland had impressed the Cragmor trustees and the institution's medical advisory board, was appointed the new house physician. A young woman named Miss Bales (her first name fails to appear in the records) was transferred to Cragmor from Clifton Springs Sanatorium to serve as the new head nurse.

But by far the most crucial change to occur at Cragmor was the naming of three medical directors to oversee the late Dr. Solly's unfledged empire: Henry W. Hoagland, Charles Fox Gardiner, and Will Howard Swan. This triumvirate of physicians, among the best medical practitioners the West had to offer, was a godsend for the institution's orphaned state. They conducted Cragmor's affairs for four unprofitable years during the odd moments they could spare from their medical practices in town. And they worked well together. Each in his own way made a distinctive contribution to the growing reputation of the sanatorium.

Henry Williamson Hoagland (1876–1942), the first of the directors named, claimed many years later to have been Palmer's personal choice to replace Solly. Hoagland's tubercular patients were few in number, so he asked Gardiner and Swan to go in with him. "We had no patients referred to Cragmor, so we had to take over our own good patients out of our private practice, put them in Cragmor where it was thirty dollars a week, which included medical attention."[4]

Hoagland had come to Colorado Springs from New Jersey at the age of ten, accompanying his tuberculous mother. As a boy of fourteen he drove the town herd through the back alleys that ran down the middle of each block. "In those days," he related, "almost everybody kept a cow and it was my job to ride up the alleys, open the corral gates, let the cow out from each lot and drive them out east of town and let them eat all day. . . . Late in the afternoon I would bring them all back to town and put each cow in its corral."[5] At sixteen Hoagland attended Colorado College, then transferred to Pennsylvania to complete his education, graduating thirteenth in a class of 333. In 1900 he returned to Colorado Springs to practice medicine. Before sharing the directorship of Cragmor with Gardiner and Swan, Hoagland had worked on the staff of St. Francis, Glockner, and Bethel hospitals.

Young Dr. Hoagland was a strong advocate of the curious treatment known as "stuffing." It consisted of dispensing mammoth portions of food, principally meat and eggs, to emaciated consumptives, hoping thereby to reduce the fever and fatten their wasted frames. Hoagland believed, as did many physicians of his time, that eating voluminously was a reliable companion cure for tuberculosis, along with fresh air, sunshine, and rest. Any pale, hacking invalid who entered his office was certain to depart on a regimen worthy of gorging the scrawniest creature back to full health. "I had one little woman," the doctor wrote, "who came from a prominent family in Chicago. . . . She was only about five feet two. I got her up to eating twenty-eight raw eggs a day. She recovered and went to Chicago—despite the twenty-eight eggs."[6]

The second new director, Charles Fox Gardiner (1857–1947),

brought to Cragmor a racy flamboyance tempered with solid medical confidence. His life as a hinterland physician was by itself a strong attraction. Patients were awed by his tales of battling Indians to deliver a baby, riding horseback 174 miles to perform a critical operation, and rescuing trappers lost in the wilderness. Gardiner helped to open up the back country with a surgeon's kit and a knapsack full of medicine.[7]

He was born in New York City, studied in Europe, and received his medical degree in 1882 from Bellevue Hospital Medical College. Like Solly, Gardiner promoted Colorado's curative climate. Soon after moving to Colorado Springs he began to specialize in the treatment of tuberculosis, wrote his first book, *Care of the Consumptive,* and coauthored an influential paper entitled "Colorado Springs Region as a Health Resort."

Gardiner was also a resourceful businessman. For several years he developed and sold at great profit the tent that bore his name. Indeed, many outdoor sanatoriums, including Nordrach Ranch and the later Modern Woodmen of America, based their appeal on the canopied or frame-sheltered dwelling known popularly as the "Gardiner Sanitary Tent." Several of those first canvas structures preceded Gardiner to Cragmor. His tents dotted the landscape whenever lungers needed lodging before comfort.[8]

This pioneer doctor lived a long, eventful life. He still actively practiced medicine at seventy-nine years of age. At eighty-one he published a best-selling autobiography, *Doctor at Timberline.* When he died in 1947 at the ripe old age of eighty-nine, Gardiner was eulogized as the city's most beloved physician.

As Hoagland brought his fetish for food to Cragmor's inmates, so Gardiner conveyed the blessings of outdoor living. His tents were designed in an octagonal shape to allow a maximum supply of fresh air to circulate freely, swirling through the interior and into the patient's lungs no matter what the weather was like on the other side of the canvas. Dr. Gardiner's daughter was among the many detractors who disdained her father's fresh-air philosophy. Speaking of his patients at Woodmen, who spent many winter days seated in a snowbank outside her father's tents, she reports that "they sat there with rugs over their legs and nearly froze to death. It was agony for them. I would say to my father, 'I'd rather die with tuberculosis tomorrow than sit out there!' He'd reply, 'Oh, but fresh air means so much!' It didn't mean a thing. The 'well' person wouldn't have dreamed of sitting outside in such inclement weather.' "[9]

His daughter's criticism failed to deter Gardiner with his tent enterprise. Neither did the wind. When it blew the tents down, he would simply reconstruct them with partial wooden sides and a wooden floor. When patients complained of the cold, he would dispense another blanket, along with warm words of encouragement. And thus Cragmor, for as long as eight years and through the instigation of Charles Fox Gardiner, enjoyed a taste of the same portable canvas life that had brought both shelter and great discomfort to numerous lungers throughout the Pikes Peak region.

The third gentleman to assume command of the renovated institution was Will Howard Swan (1867–1932), one of General Palmer's private physicians. Swan was one of the most congenial and capable doctors in the area. For nearly thirty months he was at the beck and call of Palmer, whose illness often required his personal assistance at Glen Eyrie. His other patients—the consumptives—were treated at Cragmor.

One of Swan's patients, John J. Lipset, had come to Colorado Springs when told by his doctor in North Carolina that he was dying of tuberculosis. As soon as he met Will Swan, he knew he had come to the right place and the right man. "If I should die," he wrote, "I would die in kind and competent hands." Lipset wrote the following tribute to Swan: "Dr. Swan was a most distinguished tuberculosis specialist, a successful physician respected by his confrères and beloved by his patients, a delightful dinner-companion and conversationalist, a friend to be proud of. A great-hearted, modest, good man, he wished for no connection with formal religion, but he was loved and admired by priests, professors, and prostitutes."[10] Together with Hoagland's love for food and Gardiner's relish for fresh air, Will Swan contributed that rare and wholesome ingredient to curing all ills: an abiding affection for the patients he served.

Cragmor neither flourished nor floundered under the regency of Hoagland, Gardiner, and Swan. They merely kept the place going, exuding good will, dispensing medical aid, and enriching the lives of the few convalescent lungers who were irregularly admitted to "Edwin Solly Sanatorium," the name Swan once insisted should prevail over the more widely used Cragmor. They held Cragmor intact for four years, struggling to break even. In the end, though, they had to give it up; the financial strain was too much. Their own respective practices in town had suffered and the sanatorium had become a philanthropic rather than a profit-making venture. They agreed among themselves that the time was ripe for a permanent director to enter the scene. Gardiner hoped he would be a man of unswerving altruistic ideals. Hoagland prayed he might build Solly's proposed Sun Palace. And Swan expressed the desire that he might expand the facilities that Solly had so deeply cherished. All three concurred that whoever came to foster grandeur at Cragmor would face an enormous challenge.[11]

He upon whom this new investiture fell was himself a rehabilitated consumptive from Virginia. Alexius M. Forster was twenty-three years old and fresh out of medical school when the Great White Plague assaulted his frame. By the time he was admitted to Saranac Lake Sanatorium to seek Dr. Trudeau's famed open-air rest cure, Forster had wasted away to 114 pounds and had a fever of 104 degrees. With just over one hundred dollars in his pocket, he soon became a charity case at Saranac. Many years later, when reflecting upon that experience, Forster remarked, "As my clothes wore out I was outfitted with garments of those who had died."[12]

Dr. Trudeau, a feisty, self-assured little man, gave Forster part-time work at Saranac helping fellow consumptives cope with their misery. Within a year the young doctor was well enough to accept a medical assistantship at the Gaylord Farm Sanatorium in Connecticut. For nine months he taught a course without pay at the nearby Yale Medical College, which enabled him then to secure a minor teaching position at Johns Hopkins Medical School for four years (1906–1909). Meanwhile, he served as resident physician of the Eudowood Sanatorium at Towson, just outside of Baltimore, Maryland, a charge that he fulfilled with such devotion and imagination that in 1908 he was awarded a gold medal at the International Tuberculosis Congress in Washington, D.C.

Forster's presence at this ITC gathering was especially significant for the future of Cragmor. There he met Gerald Webb of Colorado Springs, the man who would later persuade him to buy the unmanaged institution that Solly built. Webb was intrigued by Forster's work at Eudowood, a rural farm colony located among the placid lakes and fertile fields of the Maryland countryside. The center was a self-sustaining farm colony under Forster's sole supervision. It consisted of about one hundred acres of arable land—approximately the same size as Cragmor—and paid its way by employing patients as farmhands. It was Forster's thesis that agriculture represented the best form of exercise for the tuberculous, both from a therapeutic and an economic standpoint.[13] Forster's success with that outdoor community of consumptive farmers so impressed Gerald Webb that upon his return to Colorado Springs he spoke glowingly of Forster to his medical colleagues, thus laying the groundwork for the young doctor's future appointment at Cragmor.

On his part, Forster was learning more and more about Colorado Springs, Cragmor, and its founder Edwin Solly, whom he greatly admired. Indeed, he treasured his dog-eared edition of Solly's *Medical Climatology* up to the day he died. He had also read Charles Denison's *Rocky Mountain Health Resorts* (1880) and he frequently quoted from other writings by noted Colorado physicians.[14]

In addition, in the fall of 1907 Forster had become more directly aware of the Pikes Peak region and its celebrated virtues as a winter health resort through Dr. A. F. McKay. This intrepid public relations man conducted an amazing one-man advertising campaign on behalf of Colorado Springs up and down the East Coast for over ten months.[15] When he stumped into Baltimore, Forster encouraged his students at Johns Hopkins to join him one evening for McKay's presentation. The Colorado doctor's most effective tool of persuasion was a pamphlet of some ninety photographs which he himself had taken, each representing a different day of the winter months. Each snapshot had been taken at the same hour each day with the same subject in the background: the towering, snow-capped hump of Pikes Peak. McKay had attached to each photograph the weather report and meteorological tables corresponding to that winter day. The album was intended, of course, to overpower his audience with living proof of the late Edwin Solly's contention that Colorado Springs was the superlative paradise on earth for consumptives, the sun capital of the world. That Forster too became an eager convert to McKay's engaging panegyric on the City of Sunshine is well attested by his purchase, within three year's time, of 110 acres of sun-blessed sanatorium soil right in the heartland of Pikes Peak.

Forster found another source of information on Colorado Springs—and Cragmor in particular—about this same time. While Drs. Gardiner, Hoagland, and Swan were attempting to operate the sanatorium on a break-even basis, Thomas MacLaren, Solly's indefatigable architect, was still imbued with ideas about building the Sun Palace. Despite Solly's recent death, MacLaren had continued to design and redesign the monumental structure that he and Cragmor's founder had first envisioned several years earlier. MacLaren went so far as to submit several impressive sketches of the proposed main building to the *American Architect and Building News*, an influential Boston journal. Some of those sketches, together with MacLaren's accompanying article about Cragmor, the Nordrach Ranch, and the notorious Gardiner tent, were reprinted in the September 1908 issue of the *Brickbuilder*, another Boston journal devoted to the interests of innovative architectural design.[16] Such pronouncements made a solid impact on the sanatorium world of the eastern seaboard; moreover, they provided Alexius Forster with graphic insights into the Solly-MacLaren sun porch concept, as well as his first visual perception of the mammoth structure that it would one day be his task to build, modify, or scuttle.

Gerald Webb and other Colorado physicians distributed reprints of the MacLaren article far and wide. It became a prime piece of propaganda at medical conferences to promote sleeping porches, open-air treatment, and the Gardiner tent. Eastern architects requested copies of the plans, specifications, and general arrangement of the proposed building. Although not yet built, the Cragmor Sun Palace was endorsed as "a model to be followed in building new sanatoriums in the eastern states."[17]

Soon after the circulation of the MacLaren article, Colorado Springs was chosen as the site of the 1909 National Tuberculosis Exhibit from Washington D.C. The conference began in late October and featured periodic lectures, demonstrations, displays, debates, and public forum discussions that ran over a four-week period of time. Thousands of people attended the programs, many from out of state. One visitor in the crowd was Alexius Forster. At last he had a firsthand glimpse of Cragmor, a first look at Pikes Peak, and his first impression of a lively western town. Webb made a special point of introducing him to Drs. Gardiner, Hoagland, and Swan and then spent half a day showing him about the Cragmor facilities.

According to Forster's 1909 journal, there had never been anything quite like that colorful Colorado consumption conference. The governor blessed the event by declaring November 1, 1909, "Antituberculosis Sunday" throughout the state.[18] All churches were encouraged to campaign against the dreaded disease, and on Monday school classes above the sixth grade were dismissed to allow young people to attend the midtown displays and special events. The streetcar company even agreed to furnish free transportation for out-of-town pupils.

The symposium began as a sober medical conference, intended for studied enlightenment, but by the end of the third week many of the activities were beginning to degenerate into a kind of Wild West roadshow of open-air squabbles and unruliness. A carnavalesque atmosphere enveloped many of the proceedings at the Durkee Building. Banners, streamers, and posters decked the auditorium where nightly programs and daily exhibits were held. Some unscheduled soapbox orators interrupted the more staid and formal presentations to clamor for the elimination of the public drinking cup and to insist that the telephone company disinfect all public phones daily. One irate layman shouted for the prohibition of open-air markets where fruits and vegetables were displayed. "There they are," he cried, "collecting all the dust that blows and all the bugs in the dust!"[19]

Tensions mounted. A street fight broke out when those who loudly vied for increased sanitary measures to protect the community from infection encountered a hostile reception from the camp that favored driving the dirty lungers out of town. Some quick police action and low-key press coverage averted adverse publicity.

Bitterness was not confined to the ordinary laypeople. Invited speakers radiated antipathy as well. Father William O'Ryan, pastor of St. Leo's Church in Denver, for example, in a dramatic and uncharitable keynote address demanded that all infected lungers "learn to observe established rules of hygiene or get the hell out of town." He reminded the fifteen hundred people in attendance at his lecture that Colorado Springs now had the reputation of being "the most contagious city in America." He pounded on the podium: "If you hackers won't learn the common rules of sanitation and decent conduct, then kindly remove yourselves from among us." Another major speaker echoed the same sentiment. James H. Pershing, president of the Associated Charities of Denver, insisted that the community wanted its invalids but with reservation: "They're good for business, but we must make them observe proper rules," he said. Pershing too deplored coughing and spitting on the city streets. He concluded his talk asking for the strict enactment of laws against that old nasty practice of "promiscuous expectoration."[20]

It took only four or five such speeches to convert a dignified national exhibit into a circus show. One quarrel splashed out from Durkee Hall onto the street below, involving a Dr. James C. Ross, who vigorously opposed the classification of tuberculosis as a communicable disease, against a louder foe representing the state department of health, a Mr. Fisher, who yelled back at Ross that consumption was the most infectious of all ailments. The two gentlemen and their coteries were so adamant in shouting their views that they were all cited for disturbing the public peace.[21]

The quacks, too, laden with their blessed potions, serums, and magical inhalers, paraded merchandise through the parks and on the street corners. Faith healers gathered to denounce medical treatment; physicians reproached charlatans; politicians spewed invectives; consumptives coughed; and little children giggled with glee over the blessed good fun of it all.

The convention terminated with the formulation of new regulations to improve sanitary conditions and, with the city council's approval, to require the registration of all resident tuberculars. Some of the extreme measures that anticonsumptives had advocated failed, such as the effort to oblige lungers to wear bells around their necks.[22]

The "Pukers Parley," as one young wag dubbed the consumptive conference, was a dramatic way of introducing Alexius Forster to his future home. How much of the pageantry and fuss he actually took in we know only from his sketchy but colorful journal notations, but he could not have left without carrying away a distinct impression that here indeed was a town whose citizenry responded intensely to the disease that for many ages had reigned as the major destroyer of young lives throughout the world. More than eight thousand individuals had viewed the Durkee Building exhibit alone. It was the largest public turn-out for an organized indoor event in the history of Colorado Springs.

It was shortly after the conference that Drs. Gardiner, Hoagland, and Swan began to manifest feelings of disenchantment over their task of governing Cragmor. In fact, upon learning of the death several months earlier of William J. Palmer (March 13, 1909), Hoagland had announced his intention to give up his post within a year's time and return to private practice. It was principally out of deference to a deathbed request from Palmer that he stayed on as long as he did. In point of fact, Cragmor was becoming a financial albatross. Though filled to its meager capacity, particularly after October of 1909 when its rates were substantially reduced, the institution was not impressively solvent. On this account, and because all three directors agreed that the sanatorium warranted the presence of a full-time administrator who had no medical commitments elsewhere, it was amicably decided in January of 1910 to sell the Cragmor property.

Initially, however, because several community residents feared misappropriation of Solly's original intentions if Cragmor were sold to an outsider, the asylum stayed in local hands. Joel Addison Hayes, president of the First National Bank, believed that Cragmor was too great an asset to place it on the open market. He therefore persuaded four of his business associates to join him in an effort to keep the place going.[23]

Now Hayes needed to find a resident medical director. Neither Gardiner, Hoagland, nor Swan wanted the job. Hayes's personal choice was his own son-in-law, the convivial English physician Gerald B. Webb. An excellent choice indeed! Webb was prominent in the public eye, esteemed in the best social circles for his sportsmanship, decorum, and talent, distinguished internationally as an authority on tuberculosis, and beloved by his patients for his winsome bedside manner and personal charm. But Webb did not want the job either. He said he was much too busy to run Cragmor with his downtown medical practice and his research commitments. But he also said that such a task was perfectly well-suited for a fine young physician he knew named Alexius M. Forster.

Hayes and his opulent friends, while initially disappointed to have Webb turn down their offer, deferred to the recommendation. None of them seemed all that interested in Cragmor's actual operation—they were only concerned with protecting their investment. They had no time to spare to run its facilities, no commitment to its clientele, and little patience for lungers. Thus they authorized Webb to contract with whomever he felt was best equipped to administer the asylum and, if necessary, they assured him that they would gladly give up their newly purchased interest in the place if that would entice his man to take the job.

So it was that Alexius Forster ran across Gerald Webb again, this time at a Philadelphia medical conference in the early spring of 1910. Forster had recently accepted an appointment as director of two neighboring rural sanatoriums outside of Louisville, Kentucky. However, the dapper Colorado Springs physician had come to Philadelphia expressly to persuade Forster to buy Cragmor and become its resident director. Webb spotted Forster across the room at a cocktail party at the close of the conference. In a casual and elegant manner, so characteristic of this gentleman who never ventured before the public eye without a white carnation in his lapel, Webb took him aside for a friendly chat. "I think you should buy Cragmor. It's yours for the asking. A fine price." Forster thanked Webb for his generous offer saying: "We sanatorium men are not paid salaries which will enable us to buy anything more than bare necessities." But Webb mentioned his wealthy father-in-law: "I'll ask Joel Hayes to hold on to Cragmor for you, to keep it in your name, and you can pay them back as the place develops."

At the time Forster felt that Webb was simply showing a kindly professional interest in his welfare. After his return trip home to Louisville, he had almost dismissed the matter from his mind when one afternoon a month later a telegram arrived with the following laconic message: "Cragmor is yours. G.B.W." Of that startling communication, Forster wrote: "It is not hard to imagine my surprise and consternation. Only the year before I had taken a new position which presented great opportunities and I felt that my future was fixed. I immediately took the train for Colorado Springs and found that on the recommendation of Dr. Webb, Cragmor had been bought and that I was expected to come out and take charge. After a careful survey of the situation I returned home and resigned my former position."[24]

Forster, then twenty-nine years of age, took charge of the institution in the fall of 1910—its resident director and sole proprietor. Permissive freedom of movement and conduct characterized his regime from its inception. Patients were allowed full use of Cragmor's physical plant and natural surroundings. Though assigned to specific quarters, they were encouraged to socialize without fetters and to cohabit with discretion. Another feature of Forster's policy was to open the sanatorium to other physicians, who were permitted to treat their patients there any time of the day or night. While technically a private institution, Cragmor maintained an open-door policy to the medical community.

The brief Solly era and subsequent regency period must have seemed like the hermetic Dark Ages to the liberated clientele and nursing staff of this renascent Cragmor. Whereas Solly had been disposed to dismiss any rule-breaker perfunctorily, Forster, seemingly unruffled by the miscreant or frivolous dandy in his presence, absolved wayward deeds and made allowances for unruly behavior—at least during the first fifteen years or so of his rule. Whereas Hoagland has insisted on a controlled program of gorging the patient with high-protein foods, Forster relaxed mealtime rigidity, encouraged a more open and convivial atmosphere in the dining room, and broadened the bill of fare to include pastries, fruits, and wine. And whereas Gardiner had obliged his patients to withstand the rigors of winter in those celebrated tents, Forster ordered the gradual removal of all mobile canvas housing from the Cragmor property. He had no quarrel with the fresh-air philosophy; indeed, he often stated that no one had been able to improve on the Solly-MacLaren sleeping porch idea.[25] Yet his focal point was different. The Forster philosophy of health care emphasized physical comfort and mental buoyancy above everything else. Whereas Will Swan, the modest and unassuming healer, had attended his patients according to prescribed canons of strict medical practice,

Forster was often indulgent, uncommonly relaxed, and generally unconcerned about propriety and rules.

In short, Forster fostered a spirit of epicurean delight and gladsome unrestraint at Cragmor. Medically he fully endorsed Solly's affirmation that "fresh air, sunshine, and good food in a sanatorium regime was the most salutary approach for treating tuberculosis,"[26] but he added to Solly's pronouncement his own inimitable dash of tolerance for social levity. High mountain living became high life in the mountains. In due course Forster's Cragmor was known throughout the sanatorium world for its bounteous, free-swinging liberality. Its name became synonymous with luxury and ease: Cragmor, the pleasure dome for wealthy chasers; the rules-free refuge for the sick-in-lung but light-of-heart; the bacchanalian haven for carefree convalescents, handsomely equipped to monitor any symptom of the Great White Plague in its warm-blooded gallants and fevered maidens.

While an ambiance for fun and games was in gestation on Cragmor Bluff, the city was undergoing another round of social discord over public fears of contagion. Old battle lines were drawn anew between negligent pukers and irate anticonsumptives. The catalyst for this most recent outbreak of contention was the enactment of a radical public health measure intended to embarrass or shame careless lungers. Health officials required "the examination of the dust of street cars and sputum spots" throughout the city in an effort to identify wanton tubercle bacilli "and to report findings in the daily papers . . . as a means of enforcing the ordinance relative to expectorating in street cars and public places."[27] This formal edict was taken all too seriously by well-meaning sputum-checkers. As a result, animosities spread and tempers exploded on a scale much greater than any contagion. Anyone seen coughing or spitting in public was subject to a fine; most were subjected to verbal abuse. Pedestrians and streetcar riders were the most frequent victims of the inquisitorial mandate. Forster wrote that some "defenders of cleanliness" rode the trolleys just looking for trouble. Elsewhere, at Hibbard's Department Store an argument erupted when an officious clerk rudely insulted an elderly wheezing Christmas shopper, a woman who was merely suffering from a troublesome head cold. The clerk had mistaken her innocent discharge for the distillation of illicit sputum.[28]

Many indigent lungers continued to dwell in tents and make-shift hovels in the city parks throughout the winter months of 1910–11. These abodes too were the target of uncharitable taunts. Self-appointed vigilantes, under the guise of reforming the lungers of their nasty coughing habits, harassed them with rude gestures and homemade signs. A Menace to the Community, read one placard placed near a downtown tent settlement. No Promiscuous Mingling, read another. Segregate the Lungers, stated a third. Other haranguing was more bitter and cruel. One group of insensitive schoolchildren marched around a tubercular's tent shouting "Unclean, unclean, better dead and never seen!" as though the hapless tent dweller was a medieval leper. For their part, the consumptives countered with angry retorts: "You take our money, then expel us!" "Where else are we to live? This is our home!" "You have no right to legislate the way a person breathes!"[29]

The polemic became widely abusive by March of 1910, soon after the announcement of a two-storied, double-winged sanatorium for the needy sick. The institution, named Sunnyrest, was proposed by the Board of Associated Charities to take in patients at no more than five dollars weekly. "Any patient who can afford to pay six dollars will be asked to do so," stated one of the board members, "and those who are entirely without funds will be cared for gratis." The purpose of the enterprise, insofar as the Springs was concerned, was to move indigent consumptives off of the city streets and out of unsanitary local tents and shacks. A laudatory idea, but it precipitated trouble when several peevish residents on East Boulder Street, whose homes were near the proposed site, raised a public furor. "Construction must cease," they demanded. "A sanatorium here will depreciate property and will be inimical from a health standpoint." When the health department refused to condemn the new proposal, the offended neighborhood residents protested more heatedly. Some homeowners hired attorneys, others filed lawsuits and a few carried placards reviling city officials and deriding the lungers. So much opposition attended the first proposed location that another site had to be found beyond the stormy fringe and the city limits.[30]

But again the same objections were raised. This time a physician led the campaign. He claimed that pupils at nearby Columbia School would be liable to infection if the sanatorium were built in that area. His warning was sufficient; no sooner did the doctor's alarm reach the press than a new wave of protests by aroused parents hit the streets. It was at this juncture that some browbeaten consumptives assembled to answer their foes. On June 10, 1910, they told a reporter, "We resent the suggestion that our presence is a menace to the health of the community." They too carried placards and then sought the support of public officials and the medical community.[31]

The following day O. R. Gillett, a public health officer, argued before the city council that lungers represented a serious health hazard to the general populace. "They should all be removed to a sanatorium," he pleaded. Within ten days the council responded, passing an important ordinance against the construction of any sanatorium or hospital for tuberculars within the city limits, their objections being based on the grounds that such an institution would prove detrimental to the health of those whose homes were located nearby.[32]

Finally the beleaguered Sunnyrest Sanatorium was built. Its long-delayed construction induced the local press to carry a joyous conciliatory headline: "Colorado Springs Has Proven Its Sense of Brotherhood."[33] Quite suddenly, the guile, rancor, and animosity had faded away.

And what did all the fuss over penniless chasers have to do with the smug and smiling affluence of Cragmor? A great deal, if we note the concern with which Forster had observed the social disturbance. To Forster, whose sympathies clearly lay with the lungers' rights to receive proper care, the problem brought into focus one forgotten aspect of Edwin Solly's old dream. It will be remembered that Solly had hoped to build a mammoth central building and to use the profits derived from its operation for the construction of a sanatorium for poor tuberculars. As the disputes over Sunnyrest mounted and Forster's concern for the down-trodden, tent-living lungers increased, he realized that Solly's plan for a Sun Palace, once intended only for the upper crust of society's numerous consumptives, could be modified to provide medical service for destitute patients as well. Forster saw thereby the possibility of ameliorating a serious social conflict, reducing local squabbles, and augmenting Cragmor's revenue—all with the laying of a single cornerstone.[34]

Accordingly, it was now Forster's turn to tilt at windmills. His quiet, unheralded first year behind him, he was now ready to make his presence known. Indeed, he intended to out-Solly Solly with a plan so unique, so radical, that it would be greeted as an extraordinary wonder of the modern age. He would build a combination Sun Palace, sanatorium community, cottage resort, industrial settlement, and residential estate. He would astound the nation with an establishment of unparalleled benefit to medical science. In a word, he would build a Cragmor known at home and abroad as "the most novel sanatorium in the world."[35]

Before construction of the main building could begin, Forster needed only to turn MacLaren's plans over to a contractor. However, he decided to ignore the MacLaren version in favor of something more elaborate, awesome, expensive, and revolutionary. For reasons not apparent, he also dumped MacLaren as the architect.[36] Cragmor's new director preferred the ailing George Edward Barton as the architect of record for the new, ineffable project. Barton's main call to fame was his design of the early phase of a controversial haven for paupers known as the Myron Stratton Home.[37] But before he could complete that project, his health failed. Though he hung on for another two years before his death in 1913, Barton never completed the Stratton plan and it was reassigned to others.

One year before he was stricken, Barton was commissioned by Forster to come up with a design for "the New Cragmor." Barton literally spent himself at that task, laboring night and day to come up with a plan that would please Dr. Forster and the Cragmor association. While the toil of the enterprise may have taxed his strength, it also charged his emotional reserve with great excitement. He delved into archaeology, studied ancient architecture and sanitation, read the history of ancient Persia, pondered the traditions and designs of Indian pueblo dwellings, and investigated the lore and mystique of the Aztecs and their descendants. At last his knowledge coalesced, his readings and musings solidified, and George Edward Barton emerged from his study with an elaborate scheme of mortar, adobe, light, ventilation, and internal design. He took his plan to Forster, who received it with an ebullience reserved only for those who achieve rare beatific unions or see beyond the veil. "It is a masterpiece," Forster wrote, "a work of great magnitude; George Barton has fashioned my idea of a perfect sanatorium!"[38] Barton was delighted. He went home, collapsed, and following a protracted but unavailing convalescence, died.

In the meantime Forster launched a premature but fervid campaign to publicize his future eyrie for consumptives. He first needed to convince the always supportive Joel Addison Hayes of the First National Bank to stand behind the proposition. Hayes readily agreed to endorse the plan, but requested that William A. Otis be included in the financial arrangements. Otis had been a part-owner of Cragmor before Forster's arrival, he was now willing to stake his name and a portion of his fortune on the success of the exciting new edifice.

Forster next petitioned for the medical endorsement of his influential friend Gerald B. Webb. Had Webb demurred—and any man of common sense might well have done so—it was not for long. By early October Forster released Webb's name as his staunch supporter for "the scientific feature of the plan."[39]

It now remained his task to persuade the community at large—a skeptical citizenry that had already begun to distrust consumptives and would prefer to see them vanish from the scene, sputum cups and all. The challenge he faced was to sell Colorado Springs on the novel idea of approving a venture expected to cost over half a million dollars for the central building alone. To this end Forster wisely befriended one of the leading news people of the city, T. Wynn Ross of the *Colorado Springs Gazette*. Delighted to have a scoop for his Sunday edition, Ross wrote a glowing description of Forster's extraordinary notion, then included a photograph of Barton's clay-mold model of the proposed central plant. His enthusiastic article began with the words: "Within a year, a building will spring up that will be the first reproduction of the ancient pueblo Indians ever constructed in the world for the uses of civilized people. Colorado Springs will be famed the world over for this structure." The account then continued with superlatives and hyperbole suited to the subject: "There will be no trace of the ordinary sanatorium life. It will be a new era in the treatment of the disease. Surrounded by some of the most wonderful scenery of the region, in the midst of flower gardens [the patients] will be in the midst of a community enhanced by every available inducement to cure. The whole atmosphere will be of comfort."[40] Thus was the publicity launched. Forster had done a thorough and convincing job of indoctrination.

It was Forster's original intention to reserve one or more wings of his monstrous sanatorium for impoverished lungers but no trace of that early concern found its way into the newspaper report. On the contrary, the tenor of the first news release, elaborated in another *Gazette* article four months later, promoted the institution as the elite among sanatoriums, planned solely for the treatment of patients of means: "The men who come here will have bank accounts. . . . This is a sanatorium for wealthy invalids."[41]

At some point in all the spectacular fanfare to launch a nationwide advertising campaign on behalf of Cragmor, the notion of building a haven for the destitute was abandoned. The excitement revived instead the old saw that prestige and financial prosperity would redound to the city following the erection of a well-endowed Cragmor: "The benefit to Colorado Springs by an institution of this sort and by the patients of the means that will take treatment here is enormous. . . . The supplies for the sanatorium will be purchased from Colorado Springs merchants; the supplies for the construction will be purchased here; local laboring men will be employed . . . ," etc.[42]

Construction of the central building was scheduled for the beginning of 1913. Considerable work on smaller units was expected to be well under way by that time, including the development of a cottage community, an industrial village, and an elaborate network of pathways, gardens, arbors, reservoirs, and fountains built along the bluff. The Forster plan also included the erection of a heating plant, garage, new laundry, chapel, nurses' cottages, and tennis courts. Someone suggested that Forster's initial estimate of half a million dollars would expand by ten times that amount before the scheme was half under way.[43]

The central building was an architect's dream. Modeled after Indian pueblos, reminiscent of Mesa Verde in its finest hour, it was laid out in the form of a gigantic Maltese cross. Barton designed it to be six stories high at the center, each floor covering less space than the one beneath it. Built story upon story like a child's building-block castle, the fantastic edifice would have 150 individual suites, each room joined to a separate sleeping porch, which in turn opened out on balconies arranged like private penthouses. "A man of means," Wynn Ross reported, "can take an apartment, bring his family with him, have private tables in the dining room, take sunbaths on his own porch, and live in comfort while recovering."[44]

The most unique feature of the Forster-Barton chateau was its capacity to harness the sun. With multiple stories, porches, balconies, terraced roofs, and parlors, the whole dominion sprawling spread-eagle against the sun-baked bluff, this distinctive monstrosity, as the claim was then made, "allowed the maximum amount of sunlight to shine on eight sides of the building at once. . . . This magnificent edifice will soak in light everywhere at the same time. . . . It will be a monumental achievement to advance the treatment of tuberculosis with sunshine and fresh air."[45]

Forster also envisioned the development of health spa facilities within the building, complete with hydrothermal baths, sun parlors, and a room for gymnastics. Three elevators would run night and day. A large staff would service the needs of the guests, providing personal comfort, social amenities, the best in food, and constant medical care. Hundreds of the nation's materially blessed consumptives would find their Shangri-La reserved for them in the suite and spa sanctuary of this Maltese cross sanatorium at Cragmor's Indian pueblo resort.

But . . . like Solly's Sun Palace before it, and many utopian master plans at Cragmor since, Forster's dream flickered, sputtered, and died. By the summer of 1913 it had already been confined to oblivion: an unworkable, financially unfeasible, medically impractical, socially undesirable plan. And when that first wild frenzy of empire building had been flushed out of his system, Alexius M. Forster, M.D., was ready to settle down for a while to the mundane business of operating a modest country cure house "somewhere north of town."[46]

By now Gerald Webb may well have harbored ambivalent feelings over his choice for Cragmor's head physician. On the one hand, the young and ambitious Forster was unimpeachably efficient. He not only fulfilled his own administrative

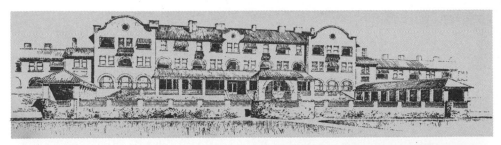

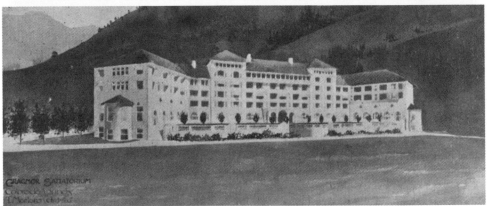

Earlier architects' dreams and schemes for Cragmor (MacLaren's two Sun Palace plans above, Barton's Maltese cross below) were never realized. The first modest dwellings hugging the bluff (upper right) opened in 1905. Later, a more substantial Main Building (lower right) was completed in October of 1914.

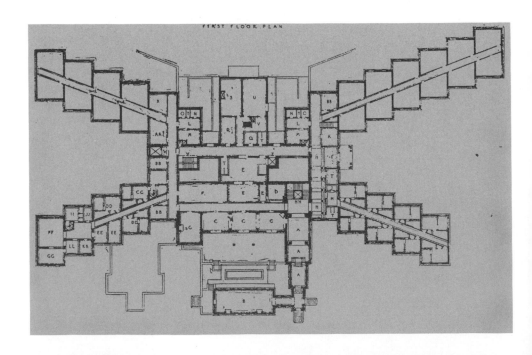

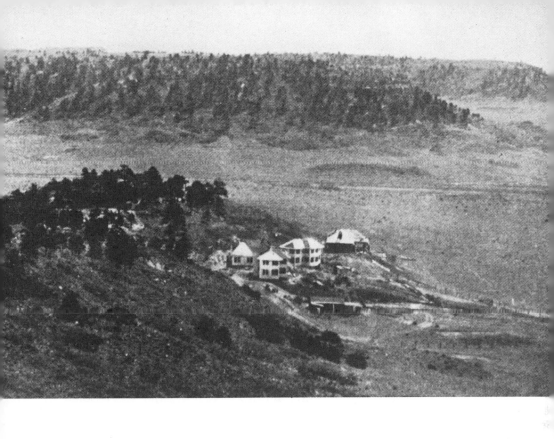

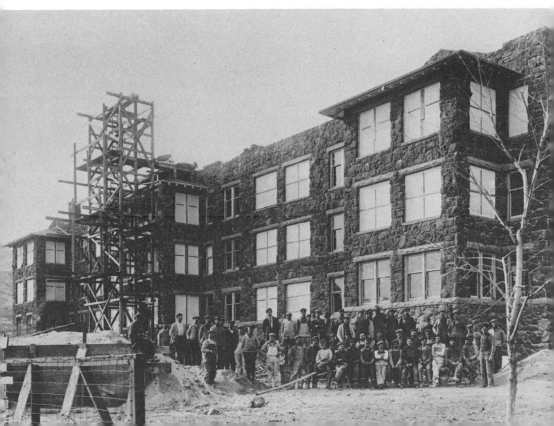

and medical duties but he also kept the books, helped with the nursing, tended to the furnaces, and even carried out cans of rubbish, sputum cups, and empty bottles to the nearby pithole. An indefatigable worker, he was up every day at dawn and was crumpled with fatigue by midnight. Nevertheless, Forster governed his sanctuary with no heed whatever to his patients' leisure-time activities. Whatever Cragmor's guests did with their spare time and bounteous reserves of cash was their business, not his, and he scrupulously practiced a policy of noninterference in their private lives.

Webb, who spent much time at Cragmor serving as the institution's major consultant, was often piqued to find in Forster's relaxed command the source for excessive frivolity among some of his own patients. He discovered, for instance, that one couple he was treating had been indulging their passions in a private cocktail tête-à-tête every afternoon, a medically improvident happy hour that gave rise to night sweats for the gentleman and a worrisome state of mind and body for the lady. Three other patients, whose respective symptoms of high fever, fatigue, and nausea had troubled Webb for more than three months, were found to be unusually fond of gambling late into the night. Upon further inquiry Webb learned that they had access to strong booze and to prevent detection they had blocked off the wholesome night air by draping dark woolen blankets over their windows, sealing in the light. One thirty-year-old lunger, a Syrian merchant whose chronic condition had stabilized during his first five months in residence, suddenly suffered a severe hemorrhage and nearly bled to death while trying to convey a large chair from the veranda of the administrative cottage to the green below. Webb was especially annoyed to walk in on yet another patient, a civil engineer from Belfast, who had converted his bathroom into a darkroom for the development of photographs; and on another, Archie Johnson from Ontario, who was just lighting a highly inflammable alcohol stove in the middle of his sleeping porch. Rest hours were not being observed; damage to fixtures, furnishings, and walls was inordinate; and patients were not always retiring at night to the same rooms where they had slept the night before.

On these accounts Webb chided the young director, suggesting to him in the strongest terms that Cragmor cease building the image of an amusement park and restore its more honorable status as a health resort. Forster countered with the argument that forms a leitmotif of his writings: "Our guests are happy. . . . Contentment is an essential ingredient for proper treatment." Webb's response, according to Forster's own brief summary of their confrontation, was as follows: "G.B. said people worn out, too much socializing, dancing."

In short, Forster's stress on "mental buoyancy" was, in Gerald Webb's opinion, an invitation to hemorrhage—"victims of walled-in pus and weekend bleedings," as Webb graphically described it. He told Forster that insofar as his own patients were concerned, he would no longer countenance any deviation from reasonable social conduct. He also reminded Forster that henceforth the director must assume full responsibility for the institution's reputation.[47]

Forster was nettled by the criticism but out of deference to Webb's concerns he promised to change the image of the place. Within twenty-four hours he circulated a memorandum to all patients, nurses, and staff, enumerating several grievances. He then posted in every cottage a list of some thirty-five rules and regulations, each edict intended "to ensure the comfort and well-being" of the patients.[48] At a special meeting called at the end of an afternoon lawn party, he asked that all guests adhere strictly to the new precepts. That the pampered lungers of Cragmor found these pronouncements more amusing than solemn may well be inferred from the fact that, in general, their festive lifestyles abated in intensity but little over the next twenty years.

With time Forster himself became more rigid and conservative, but until that gradual transformation took place, his patients remained, as a rule, a freewheeling prodigal lot. Cragmor's clientele had more money than all of the physicians attending them would ever see in a lifetime. Most of them, especially the young eastern aristocrats who had come to the resort during the first decade of Forster's regime, regarded a sanatorium as more than a serene retreat for chasing the cure. It provided them with the locale, time, and stimulation to pursue neglected hobbies, to enjoy modified recreation, to consort with members of the opposite sex, and to indulge personal whims. However, those who had been accustomed to a fast lifestyle when healthy now found that revelry or intemperance of any kind was an improvident risk, if not a threat to their very lives. Of the seventeen patients who died at Cragmor between 1911–15, more than half were said to have precipitated their demise through willful dissipation.

Forster's nonchalance, of course, was the product of a long-coddled philosophy of "live and let live," not the result of any lack of solicitude for his patients' welfare. His lenient views tended, no doubt, to encourage frivolity despite an outward display of restrictive rules. There were also those who felt that their overly tolerant director was himself a part of the problem. At thirty-one years of age Forster was still single and unattached, a strikingly handsome man of slight build, dark complexion, and a trim mustache; a dashing fellow, one would say, well-liked among the ladies and given to a basic view that most patients would recover their health if left alone to enjoy life's sweetest pleasures.

This outlook ran counter in every way to the more fastidious and eminently delicate views of the British doctor Gerald Bertram Webb. Proper deportment and decorum were the hallmarks of Webb's public and private life, and he saw little to admire in the image of license and merrymaking espoused by his younger colleague. The unassuming but accomplished and courtly Gerald Webb, long before he became a naturalized American citizen, was already recognized among the country's leading researchers in the energetic antituberculosis campaign of the early 1900s. He had come to the Colorado Rockies in 1893, aged twenty-two, accompanied by his ailing wife Jenny, hoping that the region's famed climate would improve her health. But consumption had taken its toll of her strength; she languished and died ten years after their arrival.

Webb remarried in July of 1904. His bride was Varina Howell Davis Hayes, the lovely daughter of Joel Addison Hayes, the banker. Many a young lass sighed over her loss when Webb married the radiant granddaughter of Jefferson Davis. Webb was a striking figure, tall, handsome, and athletic. Never once did he allow his mellifluent British accent to become tainted by "Little London's" western American drawl, nor did he relinquish the modest English reserve that characterized his demeanor, dress, and manners. He wore finely tailored Bond

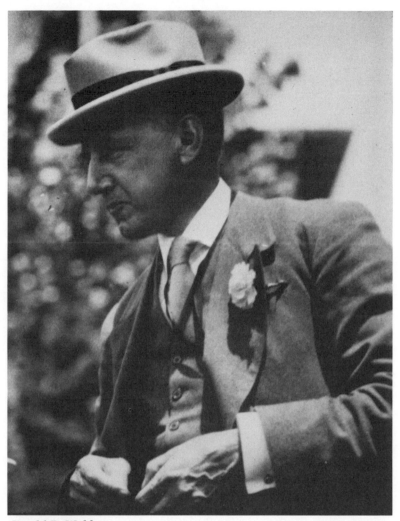

Gerald B. Webb

Street clothes, sported a carnation in his lapel, and walked
with the assurance of an ambassador who is fed on ambrosia
and favored of the gods.

Once, while attending a patient at Cragmor, Webb looked up
to see four young nurses looking on. "I don't believe this case is
all that grave to warrant such an audience," he remarked. The
nurses, a bit flustered, dispersed. "Doctor Webb," said his patient, "it isn't *my* condition that interests those young women.
. . . It's *your* presence here in *my* room!"[49]

Webb was as remarkable a sportsman as he was an eminent diagnostician. He enjoyed a solid reputation as one of the best polo and cricket players in the western United States.[50] His wizardry at chess was legendary; on one occasion he came very close to defeating the world chess champion during a match at the El Paso Club. He likewise excelled at tennis, won a statewide bridge tournament, hunted for mountain lions with President Theodore Roosevelt, and gained more than a dabbler's expertise in such fields as botany, ornithology, and paleontology. One of his favorite pastimes was participating in amateur theatricals; he welcomed any opportunity to perform Shakespeare or Shaw in local productions.

Above all, Gerald Webb was a consummate and highly distinguished physician-scholar. His biography on Rene Theophile Hyacinthe Laennec, who invented the stethoscope, was called by medical historians "the most authoritative memoir on Laennec in the English language."[51] His book on Henry Sewell, written in collaboration with Desmond S. Powell, merited a complimentary review in the *New York Times* of April 20, 1947. Webb also helped to promote and establish Cragmor's celebrated fortnightly journal and became one of its regular contributors, publishing articles that ranged from carefully researched biographies on major artists, composers, and literary figures who had lived with consumption, to a series of seventeen essays on the subject of heliotherapy.[52] "Gerald Webb was a modern-day humanist," said Maxine Sain, a former nurse. "He did as much to heal the mind and spirit as he did the body." He was as much at home with topics of philosophy, language, and literature as he was conversant about the best vintage of wines or exotic flora and fauna. Marshall Sprague wrote that Webb "taught the town not only how to drink French wine but how to pronounce the chateau bottlings properly."[53]

But tuberculosis was his central concern. For the general public he wrote two engaging books on the subject,[54] while for his colleagues of medicine he advanced new knowledge from research.[55] He brought major physicians to Colorado from all over the world, including Charles Boissevain from Holland who served as Cragmor's bacteriologist. In 1924 he founded the Colorado Foundation for Research in Tuberculosis, one of the world's first institutions to stress antimicrobial cures for phthisis.[56] He was still serving as president and research director when he died at the age of seventy-eight.

Imbued with enthusiasm to explore through research the rampant horrors of consumption, Webb turned down his father-in-law's offer to superintend the Cragmor Sanatorium when offered. Yet for over twenty years he spent many long hours of his medical career at Cragmor, attending to the needs of hundreds of tuberculous patients who had come to the institution on the strength of his reputation as its foremost consultant.[57]

From the first day of his labors at Cragmor, Webb engendered a tone of quiet sophistication and respectability in the free-wheeling asylum. Initially he found evidence of far too much riotous behavior and unchecked physical activity. Patients were cooking in their rooms, playing ball and croquet on the green, racing motorcars, riding horseback, and fraternizing late into the night. Many of his own patients who had come from the East were showing greater signs of exhaustion than of recovery. Webb soon made it clear to Forster that the health of Cragmor's guests was impaired by all the frolicking hedonistic acrobatics taking place and that the institution's restless fops and swinging flappers must return to their own beds and pursue a rigorous regimen of constant postural rest. "Dr. Webb was very stern with us," reported one of his former patients of that holiday era. "One day he took hold of my arm as I was running down the hallway in my pajamas. 'Young man, do you want to recover your health?' he asked. I was surprised by the earnestness of the question. Dr. Webb looked straight into my eyes while he spoke. 'Yes, sir. Yes, I certainly do,' I mumbled. 'Then turn around and go back to your room. Go to bed and stay there for six months!' Saying that, he turned and walked away. I went back to my bed and I stayed there for six months. Lord, there was something about that man that commanded respect."[58]

Webb brought diversion into the life of the invalid who faced the wretched task of persevering for months in a state of physical immobility. While insisting on the supreme importance of bed rest, he never once allowed a patient the luxury of mental stagnation. It was not unusual to see him enter a patient's room armed with books of classical and modern literature, nature study, or astronomy. "He first introduced me to Hazlitt," avows one grateful former paitent, "then to the reading of my temperature!"[59] Webb believed in the value of mental quietude, the healing force of positive thinking, and the tonic potency of good literature. "There are many times," he once wrote, "when it is incumbent on the wise physician to prescribe, not a posset or a purgative, but an essay or a poem."[60]

"Gerald Webb made it a point to familiarize himself with the literary interests of his patients," said one of Cragmor's former physicians.[61] One Cragmorite was alarmed to find all of his "prurient periodicals" missing. "Dr. Webb removed my cheap magazines and dime novels," he exclaimed. "I was very angry and was about to ring for the nurse when in walked the doctor with an armful of leather-bound books. He handed me a biography of Ruskin, a collection of essays by Emerson, and some poems by Tennyson. 'Here, enjoy these!' he said. 'I'll be by in a few days and we'll talk about them.' Gerald Webb was more than a doctor; he was a teacher."[62]

Another of Webb's patients was on a particularly difficult rest regimen. "The lights of Broadway had been her only joy," he recorded. One morning he found her watching a garden spider at work; for the first time in many days she seemed to show some interest in something. He informed her that the females of some species devour their husbands after the nuptials. "My," she exclaimed, "that's just like life back in New York!" Webb went on to explain that some spider mothers give their infants daily sun baths. The woman was soon intrigued. "She forgot her self-pity and turned to the study of nature," he wrote. On his next visit he brought her Thomson's *Ways of Living*, Lord Grey's *The Charm of Birds*, and F. W. Gamble's *The Animal World*. The books became her daily diet and instilled in her a renewed interest in living.[63]

Yet another protégé of Webb's reading program was a lovely young woman named Laura Jones. Thanks to Webb she became so fond of books that she cut out pictures, illustrations, and quotations and pasted them on her wall. This habit amused Webb but upset Forster. One winter when it was extremely cold and Cragmor was hurt by a local coal strike, Miss Jones made small fires out of the rest of the pages of her already mutilated books and kept herself comfortable, much in the romantic tradition of the shivering poet in *La Bohème*. That winter she read and burned an entire set of Balzac, most of Kipling, and many modern authors. Her torrid reading pace continued for five years—though the book burning ceased. Webb, in fact, had difficulty keeping her supplied with enough literature. She helped form an exclusive reading club at Cragmor, was conversant about medical findings, criticized modern poetry, and eventually recovered and left for New York. Within a year she was the hit of a Broadway production, playing the lead under the name of Laura la Tille.[64]

It was Gerald Webb's firm conviction that "the mind, like the body, will thrive best on a mixed diet, and he who experiences the variety of a number of literary forms will derive from his reading a satisfaction free from the dangers of ennui."[65] One of his former patients claims that she profited more from her half year's confinement at Cragmor than at any other time of her life: "Dr. Webb taught me to discover truths about myself hidden in great literature. One afternoon he brought me a copy of *Pickwick*. For the next six months it was Dickens, then Thackeray, than Galsworthy. . . . I was entranced! Soon I was well; they said I could go home. I was sorry to leave—that reading was the first real joy of my life."[66]

Like William Wycherly, Webb too had learned to patch pain with proverbs; each of his literary prescriptions blessed a human mind with new thought.[67] He was known to spend hours at the bedside of a chronically ill patient, discussing the value of a book or the meaning of a poem. By the magnetic charm of his personality and his genuine interest in people, Webb fomented a radical change in many lifestyles at Cragmor. The swinging sanatorium, known far and wide as a playhouse for frolicking millionaires, was given an added dimension under Webb's influence. Its sickrooms became something akin to a college of liberal arts. "I would have called it Colorado's first countryside salon!" affirmed one ex-patient.[68] His statement was not far wrong. Owing to Webb's gentle incitement, the first Cragmor lending library was established, a highly successful literary magazine was launched, and many able speakers, artists, and performers brought their talents to Cragmor. Another Cragmorite said it best: "Dr. Webb's presence was something of a renascence. He gave us culture and refinement."[69]

Webb was still serving as one of nine consultants to a greatly expanded Cragmor in May of 1931; the institution then boasted a resident staff of six physicians, one dentist, and two business managers. Later that year, however, he and Cragmor parted company for good. The pleasure-dome atmosphere had intensified during the Roaring Twenties, a matter that distressed him; some of the medical personnel were involved emotionally with their patients, a situation he found morally reprehensible; and he and the resident director had a serious dispute over an issue that he could not condone. Webb's disaffection was Cragmor's irreparable loss. He had done more to enrich and humanize the environment than any other person at any time in the institution's piquant history. Marshall Sprague, who himself was cured of tuberculosis under Gerald Webb's care at Glockner, sums up the meaning of this noble gentleman's life for many people: "Dr. Webb stood between me and the dark. He made me well, but besides that it was his gift to pass his own love of life on to me; to pass his interest in living on to me; to make me want to live as passionately as he himself wanted to live. And he did that for thousands."[70]

FOUR

Cragmor's Golden Age

Oh, Forster, how I envy you
your Colorado sunshine!
Edward Trudeau

Until the Main Building was constructed and opened in 1914, Cragmor's capacity remained at only twenty-five consumptives. Ostensibly, the admission policy before the Forster era had been nonrestrictive. When there was an opening, the previous directors had advised their colleagues in town, who in turn contacted the patients most deserving or eager to move out to the bluff. During the Forster and Webb years the practice shifted to a national recruitment effort, communicating directly with physicians in the East who had invalids waiting for a chance to chase the cure in the Rocky Mountains. Both Webb and Forster attempted to fill the guest roster with as many financially well-endowed patients as they could locate, thus bringing large sums of money to Cragmor, the community, and Colorado. By 1912, in fact, the sanatorium was admitting patients wholly on a principle of priority according to income and assets. Occupancy was customarily offered first to the wealthy, influential consumptive and then, as space allowed, to a less prosperous clientele. This remained the standard admission procedure at Cragmor until the Depression.

Forster's elitist tactics were exceedingly successful during Cragmor's early years. Many prominent and permanent citizens of Colorado Springs came via Cragmor—some with assets or investments worth millions of dollars. Other wealthy lungers came only for the cure and then moved on, but while convalescing they gave a tremendous boost to the local economy.

During Cragmor's first twelve years of operation, its patients and the institution spent an average of $300,000 per year in the community.[1] Cragmor's guests drove some of the finest custom-built automobiles made in America, wore the most fashionable clothes that money could buy, surrounded themselves with original paintings, porcelain, rare birds, and leather-bound books, dined from silver trays, hired private nurses, and conducted business by long distance calls to Wall Street.

One example among the many affluent Cragmor patients whom Gerald Webb treated was a retiring and fragile young lady of twenty-two years named Constance Pulitzer. She was a quiet girl, very ill, lacking the vivacity, stunning beauty, and plumpness of her older sister Edith, yet besting the fate of Joseph Pulitzer's first two daughters who had died of pneumonia and typhoid. Constance was chasing the cure in a private suite at the back of the Women's Cottage when her celebrated father suddenly died aboard his yacht in Savannah Harbor. Owing to the distance and her own frail condition, Constance was unable to reach New York in time for the funeral. She arrived the morning after the services were held at the fashionable St. Thomas Episcopal Church, picked up her half of the $1,500,000 joint trust her father had left his daughters, and returned to invest her fortune in several Colorado Springs business ventures. Eventually Constance recovered from tuberculosis, married the son of a British judge, and the newlyweds made their home among the elite coterie of Wood Avenue.[2]

Another luminary from the Pulitzer constellation was Arthur Billing. Ordinarily a tall and imposing gentleman, Billing arrived at Cragmor in an extremely weakened state, his huge frame stooped, his lips drawn with pain, his hands trembling. On admission Billing's fever registered 104 degrees. He was suffering from a chronic case of "galloping pulmonary tuberculosis" and a runaway affinity for alcohol. Forster struggled for six weeks drying him out and the next twenty-four months attempting to arrest the lung disease.

The son of a prominent English bishop, Billing had graduated from Cambridge and taken up drafting, then abandoned his trade to lead a wild and unrestrained life as a globe-trotting dandy. Somehow he managed to endear himself to the ailing and irascible Joseph Pulitzer, who speedily promoted the articulate Billing from a servile job as messenger to become the cantankerous publisher's private secretary. From there Pulitzer turned over a portion of the management of the *World* newspaper to Billing. Thus, before he was thirty-five, this genial and dashing Englishman had become one of the most trusted and valued members of the Pulitzer dynasty.

Pulitzer was often attracted to people for unusual reasons. One of Billing's dubious charms was his capacity to drink a prodigious amount of alcohol without showing any discernible effect. Pulitzer once derided him for bragging of this feat. Billing countered that he could consume an entire quart of champagne and no one would see any difference in his speech, carriage, or conduct. Pulitzer accepted his challenge and ordered a quart of Mumm for his braggart secretary. Billing drank the entire bottle within fifteen minutes and showed no sign of intoxication. Pulitzer was astonished and spoke often of his secretary's rare talent.[3]

Learning of Billing's skill as a draftsman, Pulitzer had sent him to Leith, Scotland, to spend a year overseeing the construction of *Honor*, Pulitzer's magnificent new yacht. Later, because Pulitzer suffered from a serious nervous disorder that made him abnormally sensitive to sound, Billing was commissioned to design a perfectly soundproof bedroom in the eccentric journalist's New York mansion. He brought all of that talent for design and innovative form to Colorado Springs where, once restored to health and pledged to abstinence, with Thomas MacLaren he engineered the construction of Cragmor's Main Building. Billing was the "unofficial" architect for the interior design of the 1914 edifice.

After two years at Cragmor, Billing could resume most of his former duties back East. Yet so enamored was he with Colorado that he returned the next summer for a fishing vacation in Estes Park. One night Forster received a call that Billing had been seriously injured in an automobile accident. He and Webb drove all night to see him, reaching Estes Park about five in the morning. They found their rehabilitated consumptive and reformed alcoholic in a critical state, his left lung pierced by a broken rib. Before an operation could be performed, Arthur Billing was dead.

Forster was keenly broken up by Billing's death. He had idolized that worldly scamp. "I never had a more loyal patient," he later wrote. "Day after day he lay in his bed and followed my instructions to the letter, not only in regard to physical rest but also in respect to his mental activity. I was only a young country doctor and I was flattered to have a patient of his ability and character submit so absolutely to my direction." It had been Forster's habit, after his evening rounds were finished, to slip over to Billing's room for a half hour chat and there he would listen in awe while Pulitzer's protégé delivered himself "in a most wonderfully entertaining fashion" on faraway lands, loose women, exotic foods, and transoceanic orgies. A close bond had been formed between the two men. His engaging friend's death left Forster empty and forlorn.[4]

Not all of Forster's first-class patients heeded his advice as religiously as Billing. Benjamin Cline resisted every service Cragmor offered. He fought the nurses, yelled at fellow invalids, and refused to listen to the doctor's orders about bed rest. Cline was a very high-strung, nervous individual. He had recently inherited two million dollars and came to Colorado Springs determined to gratify his every whim. At first he insisted on staying in a private suite at the Antlers Hotel, but later consented to drive his custom-made automobile out to Cragmor for treatment. After a week of quietude in the Men's Cottage, Cline's nervous state was still so extreme that he bolted from bed, pushing the nurse and her thermometer to the floor, ran to his car, drove downtown, and caught the first train for New York. From there he took an ocean liner to Europe. "After three or four months," Forster reported, "I had a cablegram from Switzerland saying he was coming back to follow my advice. . . . I met him at the train and found his condition so desperate that I had him taken in an ambulance to the nearest hotel where he died the next day."[5]

Of the sixty-seven patients who entered Cragmor in 1911, thirty-nine were men and twenty-eight were women. The average age was thirty for both groups. The oldest person admitted was Major Harry C. Valentine, a well-to-do lawyer from New Jersey, who died at Cragmor on the morning of his sixty-fifth day in bed and one week short of his forty-seventh birthday. The youngest invalid during Forster's inaugural years was Jack

Miller, an eighteen-year-old schoolboy from Oklahoma, whose father, it was said, owned half the Panhandle and most of Texas. The customary stay at Cragmor was about four months, although one young man remained for eleven years, while in contrast a nineteen-year-old girl committed suicide after only one night of residence.

Cragmor's initial millionaire set included the manager of a General Motors plant, a cattleman from the King Ranch, a New York financier, two accountants, a shipbuilder, three international merchants, a pair of attorneys, and several farmers who had trafficked in oil on the side.

Perhaps the most exciting character to invade Forster's tubercular haven that year was Theodore Burris from Brooklyn, New York. Under the heading marked "occupation," he signed the register as "Arizona Navajo Reservation Indian Trader." Burris, who was reared in the lap of luxury, schooled at Harvard, and apprenticed to his father's brokerage firm on Wall Street, had forsaken the easy path to a massive family inheritance and genteel wedlock by embracing a Brazilian strumpet, contracting syphilis, and becoming a slave to Scotch and rye. In January of 1911 he moved to Arizona, ostensibly to trade trunk loads of South American trinkets with the Indians, while aspiring to fulfill his doctor's firm command to dry himself out. In the course of four months' time, however, Burris nearly succumbed to myriad ailments that beset him on the reservation, among them dizzy spells, severe sweats, insomnia, chronic headaches, constant vomiting, huge welts on his backside, fissures on his tongue, the abscess of several glands, loose bowels, a partial paralysis in his arms, dreadful hallucinations, and the strange tic of having his head turn involuntarily to one side so that he found himself looking constantly over his left shoulder, unable to speak. And thus he appeared at Cragmor on May 5, 1911, a gaunt, trembling, spasmodic wreck of a man, dragging a trunk filled with useless Indian herbs, salves, and ointments. The drinking spree he had begun ten years before continued while he convalesced at Cragmor. "The patient only drinks beer when he's had too much whiskey," reported Dr. Webb. "He has everything wrong with him, yet not a symptom of TB." Burris danced by day, drank by night, sang bawdy songs to his nurses, raved at fellow patients, and was finally asked to leave the premises, uncured and incurable, labeled by Dr. Forster "a consummate nuisance and damn fool."[6]

Forster's second year saw a greater turnover among the asylum's monied chasers. Generally older, flashier, and better-endowed with wealth than their predecessors, some of the 1912 lungers caused the director a great deal of professional trouble and no small amount of personal heartache. One very ill middle-aged businessman named Richard Cole locked himself away in an upstairs room and refused to communicate with anyone. The nurse was frantic because Cole would not let her in. When she tried to force open the door, he threatened to kill himself if she entered. Forster declined to intervene, stating that "Cole will come out when he's damn good and ready." In the meantime food was left on a tray outside his room. He took it in late at night after everyone else had retired, leaving his trash and dirty linen at the door for the maid to pick up. Cole languished in solitude for twenty-seven weeks. One morning he opened the door and walked out, his face ruddy, hair combed, suitcase in hand. Forster examined him, pronounced him cured, and Cole was released. He left without a word of explanation or goodbye.[7]

An alarming emotional problem ensued when a woman, aged thirty-six, fell violently in love with her doctor. She had been discharged as cured after two months, but returned to Cragmor in June of 1912 saying that she was ill again. Several weeks later the nurse discovered that the woman was deliberately keeping her temperature up, practicing exercises of self-abuse to prolong her treatment. When the doctor paid her no heed, the patient claimed to have blood-streaked sputum, went into convulsions, and attempted to induce a hemorrhage. Still the doctor ignored her. Finally she packed her bags, stormed out of Cragmor, and returned to her husband and children in Missouri.[8]

Forster's most unsavory case that year concerned a wealthy retired farmer from North Dakota. His name was Fred Burke. Fred emitted from his breath and body the foulest stench possessed by a living mortal. Even bathing could not dispel the odor. It was so repulsive that no one on the staff could attend Fred without wretching. Finally he had to be isolated in a back cabin high on the bluff. But even then complaints were lodged, especially whenever an evening breeze carried Fred's infamous smell into the open windows of the dining area below. Forster eventually wrote to the old gentleman's daughter to come and take him back to North Dakota "to insure the well being of our other guests." After eighty-two days of Cragmor's longest and most fetid summer, Fragrant Fred departed. His cabin had to be scrubbed with lye and fumigated over a two-week period before it could be used again.[9]

That fall a teenaged schoolboy named David Arnold, reputedly worth one-quarter of a million dollars through inheritance, entered Cragmor. He was terribly frightened; his doctor back home in Arkansas had told him that he was dying of tuberculosis. His eyes were wild with fear as the nurse registered his fever: 103 degrees. David was confined to bed and lay in mortal terror of the dark. One morning a week after his admission he and his one suitcase were gone. There was no sign anywhere of David Arnold. He had simply disappeared. No one ever heard from him or saw him again.[10]

George Hogan, a thirty-one-year-old laborer from Wisconsin, entered Cragmor later that same year. He came with an advanced case of pulmonary tuberculosis and required pneumothorax immediately.[11] When it failed, the agonizing treatment was repeated. Another failure. On Christmas Eve one of the young patients in the Men's Cottage glanced up to see a body wearing a white tunic dangling on a rope outside his window. He screamed and rang for the nurse. George Hogan had tied one end of a rope around his radiator pipe, the other around his neck, and climbed out the window. He was Cragmor's second suicide that year; it did much to dampen everybody's Christmas spirit.[12]

Among the more than seventy patients admitted in 1912 only four had journeyed to Cragmor from western states. Most of the lungers were from the eastern and southern United States. They included a New York opera singer, a wholesale fruit dealer from New Orleans, and a railroad magnate from Virginia. There were six foreign invalids as well, among them John Standing, a noted physician from England and a close friend of Gerald Webb; Max Hurst, a New Jersey mercantile king who doubled his fortune by selling goods to the Russian czar; Andrés Herrera, an oil and ranching tycoon from Havana, Cuba; and Thomas P. Kennedy, whose family's money had helped to pave numerous streets in Belfast, Ireland, and build many schools in New York City.

Even without its opulent Sun Palace or its imposing pueblo castle on a Maltese cross design, Cragmor occupied center stage among the nation's sanatoriums for upper-class consumptives. An unrivaled climate and Webb's reputation brought them out; an excellent cuisine and Forster's permissive atmosphere bolstered their spirits; and superb medical attention enabled most of them to walk away to make new fortunes. By the end of 1912 Cragmor had the lowest rate of consumptive mortality for any institution of its size in the country. And Forster was especially delighted that several generous guests, grateful for the care they had received, bequeathed enough money to allow for incorporation and the construction of the long-awaited Main Building. "Cragmor will soon accommodate one hundred and fifty patients!" announced Forster as he and six associates filed articles of incorporation on January 3, 1913. "And this time," he wrote, "nothing is going to stop us."[13]

Formal incorporation took place during one of the coldest weeks ever recorded in Colorado Springs's history. While temperatures hovered near fifteen degrees below zero, Webb and Forster were warmed by the thought that as soon as the ground thawed, the institution's capitalization of $450,000, plus another $100,000 subscribed in stocks, would now permit the erection of George Edward Barton's monumental design. However, it was not to be. Notwithstanding Forster's strong objections—the one voice of dissent in the group—the board ultimately decided that Barton's design was too ambitious and costly. They voted to table the project pending further study. "We have a new corporate management," wrote Forster bitterly, "and in its first formal session it has acted with decisive haste to thwart a glorious dream."[14]

The next decision facing the board was that of finding a replacement for the deceased Barton. Webb suggested reinstating Thomas MacLaren since MacLaren's previous plan for Cragmor could be modified with no time lost and at minimal expense. Forster was still rankled over the loss of his Maltese cross chateau, but raised no objection. MacLaren was agreeable to the task, so once again the community's chief architect was engaged to engineer the construction of Edwin Solly's singular Sun Palace. The old design came out of mothballs and little Cragmor suddenly buzzed anew with the excitement of an architectural revival. For six months thereafter, Palace Plan II was coddled, toasted, and revered. MacLaren made further modifications, all downward in cost, while Forster hatched fresh visions, all on an ascending scale.

On one occasion, in late March of 1914, three bids for the construction of the Sun Palace were so satisfactorily low, so well within the amount set aside for the Main Building, that a decision was made at once to extend one of the wings beyond the original length that MacLaren had proposed. Accordingly, the lowest bidder was asked to submit an additional offer for a new section that would provide twenty additional rooms.[15] What a domain the new Cragmor was destined to be! All of the architectural hopes of the golden past were renewed. Curious citizens drove out to view the site; lumberyard and trade stores in town eagerly awaited building supply orders; plans for the ground-breaking ceremony were under way. And then . . . just as before, the $500,000 colossus just fizzled away. One week before the stone, cement, gravel, and sand could be piled on the slopes of the bluff, before the bulldozers could gouge into Cragmor's rocky terrain, before the finest showplace of America's tubercular wonderland could go up, the Cragmor board of directors met for another round of talks characterized by long faces, vacillation, and withdrawal.

Forster, understandably, was exasperated beyond words. The irony of it all left him thoroughly bemused.[16] Only one decade before, Edwin Solly had calculated that his Sun Palace would cost $200,000. Then that figure had nearly tripled with the completion of MacLaren's first plans. Later, when Barton's pueblo plan was approved, the estimated cost had soared to half a million dollars, only to climb well above five million by the time Forster had expanded the design to include a vast industrial complex. After ten long years of inflated figures, ascending quotations, and spiraling bids, all in accordance with everyone's honest effort to devise the biggest, best, and most expensive sanatorium on the planet earth, at last the time was ripe. Philanthropic gifts were pouring in. A healthy and stable corporate fund, managed by astute businessmen, was palpably available. A viable program of stock subscription was well under way, enabling local investors to reap personal returns from Cragmor's certain growth. Indeed, the institution had come of age and the prospects for the Main Building's construction were most propitious. Palatial aspirations, first espoused by Solly and now embraced by Forster, seemed to be a reality.

But the businessmen who comprised 60 percent of the board's voting power disagreed. Instead of the grandiose, multiple-winged manor, they felt it would be more prudent to ask Mac-Laren to design a modest two- to three-story building, capable of being added upon as needed. Instead of housing 150 patients, the new Cragmor, it was felt, should accommodate no more than twice its current capacity of 25 guests. And instead of spending hundreds of thousands of dollars to develop the world's largest health spa, four members of the board proposed that the initial cost outlay not exceed $80,000.

Forster was so nonplused that he considered resigning, but eventually he decided to accept the verdict of the cautious corporate directors. They had assured him, in a lengthy session convened especially to placate his anger, that as Cragmor grew and profits increased, new additions would be constructed. "Cragmor will remain a small country asylum," Forster wrote to Arthur Billing, "but, by damn, only for the present! Tomorrow, Art, we will build an empire."[17]

Meanwhile the Great White Plague rampaged unabated. A waiting list for patients hoping to enter the new Main Building was filled months before the edifice went up. And within two weeks of the structure's completion in October 1914, every room was taken.

MacLaren did a splendid job despite an 80 percent rollback in costs. His finished building comprised three stories, the first built of Colorado stone and the remaining two of concrete. Its exterior bore no resemblance to the celebrated Sun Palace I or Cragmor Palace II sketches, but followed instead a Spanish mission style that he believed was best suited to blend with the natural earth colors and vegetation of the surrounding countryside. All frills of luxury were gone, of course. No allowance was made for the lavish sun parlor, handsome billiard room, spacious reception halls, or lighted tennis courts proposed in an era of greater fantasy and illusion. But MacLaren did add a touch of elegance all his own. Running across the surface of the building's flat roof he built a three-foot wall, with numerous alcoves and sheltered corners. This gave Cragmor the only roof garden in Colorado Springs. At night it was aglow with electric lights, its recesses embellished with plants and flowers, an ideal spot for quiet dancing and cocktail parties. By day its floor was decked with reclining chairs and sun mats. In years to come Cragmor's roof garden developed into an important attraction for ebullient sun worshipers, devotees of heliotherapy.

Arthur Billing, who had remained beyond his anticipated convalescence in order to assist MacLaren, added his own special talent to the building's interior design. He spent many hours sketching labyrinthine corridors and odd-shaped suites, much to the amusement of admiring female guests. Billing gave the halls and guest rooms a touch of unique and fashionable handiwork. No two chambers were alike. A different shape, size, and dimension attended each of the twenty-eight suites. Into some Billing introduced charming fireplaces; all had a sleeping porch recess. Every corner, molding, and interior furnishing was rounded to avoid catching and holding house dust, that vexatious bane of all consumptives.

In the second-story dining hall Billing and MacLaren used a simple and inexpensive design. A large, open fireplace, built of Colorado moss rock, occupied one end of the hall, while the other end connected to a serving room, behind which were two kitchens, refrigeration units, and a cold storage plant. The dining room sported a beamed ceiling, large dormer windows opened to the west, and indirect lighting illuminated the entire hall. The area was designed to feed 150 guests. Within a decade this hall would be noted as the finest dining area in the Pikes Peak region, offering a bill of fare equal to anything served at the Broadmoor.

MacLaren adhered to the basic Solly-Forster view that Cragmor was exclusively a sanatorium for patients of means. Though considerably reduced in size from all previous architectural schemes, the Main Building still inspired visitors to remark that Cragmor was the only institution of its kind in the country. Forster echoed this sentiment in a local press release: "The rich man who contracts tuberculosis has no place else to go where he can have the personal care and attention of medical experts. There are sanatoria aplenty for the poor, but not for the

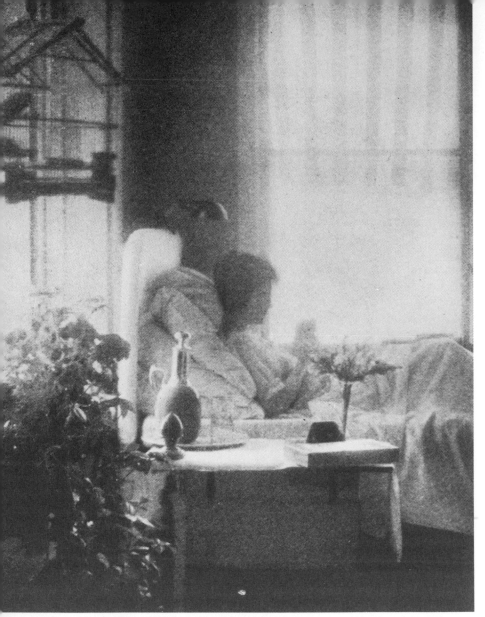

A Laura Gilpin photo, winter 1925

wealthy."[18] There was no mistaking it. Cragmor, though small, would still remain a haven for the affluent.

What was life like at Cragmor during the first year of the Main Building's operation? Had you been one of the fifty-three patients on the sanatorium's register for that year (1915), justly proud of your new central unit, enjoying the prestige of chasing the cure at one of the most important institutions for tuberculosis treatment in the country, you would have found that your daily activities were circumscribed by the seriousness of your condition. An exacting rest program greeted every invalid. While you were free to pursue your personal interests at leisure, you were constantly reminded to heed Cragmor's one rigid commandment: Thou Shalt Rest Thy Diseased Frame. "I commend my sick body into your hands," Billing had said to Forster, and that was precisely the spirit of compliance that the physicians hoped to secure from every patient.[19]

Ideally, you were among many of Cragmor's so-called incipient cases of pulmonary tuberculosis, that is, those who felt only mildly ill and whose disease stood nine chances in ten of effecting a cure within one year. If you suffered from a moderate to advanced form of consumption, you would have to count on spending from two to five years of your life in the sanatorium searching for health, and your chances might be less than four in ten of recovering. And if you did recover, the danger of relapse was as high as 50 percent.[20]

When you first arrived at Cragmor, you were put to bed for several days, so that your particular case could be studied by the medical staff. Registering a fever under one hundred degrees, you were allowed to get up. Before meals you rested in a reclining position; after meals you did the same. At other times you were allowed to read or write or visit among your companions—preferably in the open air. You were encouraged to spend a good deal of time sunbathing either on the roof garden, the front lawn, or the cottage piazza. You spent the rest hour—between two and four in the afternoon—in a horizontal position on your screened-in sleeping porch. After dinner you were free to take a stroll on any of the several walks designed for that purpose along the bluff.

You went to bed at 8:30, turned your lights out by 9:30, and slept for ten hours. You ate nourishing food three times a day. Forster was proud to report that "no effort or expense is spared in making Cragmor's table the very best."[21] Fresh milk and cream were delivered daily from the Holland Dairy and your water supply was piped fifteen miles to the sanatorium from mountain springs. With your doctor's permission you could ride one of the three or four horses maintained at the livery, though for the most part the animals were reserved for conveying the sanatorium's carriage to and from the streetcar line that linked the coal mining fields one mile to the west with the center of town four and one-half miles to the south. Cragmor also owned one automobile, and for one dollar you could ride into town. If you could afford to drive a vehicle of your own—and most of the patients did—you did so sparingly because the medical staff discouraged patients from using their own motorcars on the sanatorium property owing to the ensuing noise and dust problems. The streetcar line that connected Cragmor with downtown brought deliveries of mail and supplies twice daily.

Wherever you resided—whether in one of the twenty-eight plush suites in the Main Building, in one of the renovated cottages, in a remote hillside cabin, or in a less desirable Gardiner tent (these being reserved for the most hearty and adventuresome lungers, or for "the most foolhardy and rash," as Forster would say)—you had running water, electric lights, and a bell connected to the nurses' quarters. If you remained in a tent, you paid the lowest rate: $20 per week. The best suite in the Main Building would cost $15 more. These charges included everything: food, lodging, medical attention, general nursing, tray service, vaccines, throat treatment, etc.

If you indulged in games of chance or card playing during your spare time, no one seemed to mind, except for the fact that you did so at the peril of incurring Forster's verbal wrath, as he often pronounced strong invectives against gambling of any kind: "When I see my patients wasting a lot of time and unduly exciting themselves over bridge parties, I feel a little sense of irritation and anxiety on their account."[22] Although Forster often barked loudly in this regard, his patients soon realized that he made no concerted effort to prohibit the practice. If card playing was not your forte, you had plenty of time to read. And if Gerald Webb had anything to say about your reading habits, you read only the best books of classical literature.

While disease was a part of your everyday life, breath, and movement, you never discussed the subject with anyone except a doctor or a nurse. It was commonly understood that small talk about blood and pus and sputum and ugly gaping wounds among fellow patients was strictly forbidden. The subject of death was taboo. You were acutely conscious, of course, that people died at Cragmor. Indeed, a special room was always reserved for the terminally ill on the top floor at the southwest corner of the Main Building. For long periods of time the door to that restricted room would remain closed. Then there would be a flurry of activity—doctors, nurses, close relatives, sometimes a priest, later the coroner—and the next morning the door would be wide open and fresh air would blow in from the empty sleeping porch across the well-scrubbed sunlit room into the corridor. It was a familiar adage at Cragmor that death and the garbage were always removed before dawn. After all, Cragmor was advertised internationally for its curative function. It was hailed among the finest medical centers in the country, a place where people came to be healed, where one struggled against death and dying. There were obviously a few morbid souls among you who considered Cragmor a hospital designated for dying, who were there for the express purpose of expiring, especially when it was too awkward to die at home. But they were the exception. You tried not to think about them.

Among the convalescents were many wealthy, well-educated chasers whose company you enjoyed and whose tales about their own preconsumptive lives enriched your leisure hours. There was David Myers, a renowned portrait painter, who furthered his career and fattened his personal bank account over an eighteen-month convalescence as Cragmor's self-proclaimed artist-in-residence. There was Charles H. Small, another talented artist, himself a professional cartoonist and political satirist, who amused fellow lungers with naughty caricatures depicting their nocturnal sprees. He was a mischievous chap, wrote Forster, always on the lookout for private orgies. And there was Carlton Masters, a former shipmate of four notorious captains of the Seven Seas. He had made his fortune trafficking in the eastern slave trade and could tell heinous tales about kidnappings, smuggling, and dope rings.[23]

A few celebrities from various fields of entertainment also came to Cragmor. Murielane Pancost, the concert soprano, spent several months coughing bad notes betimes with the good. Jeanette MacCoil, a well-known New York City musician, offered Cragmorites a series of recitals as part of her brief curative visit.

Throughout the Pikes Peak region there were noted writers, artists, musicians, and actors chasing the cure. The resort city enjoyed a renown far more impressive than their collective fame. Judges and paupers alike gravitated to the clean air, clear sunshine, and high altitude of Colorado Springs, the most highly proclaimed city in America for ailing lungs. And its climate offered the perfect tonic to renew neglected creative talents. For this reason the painter Russell Cheney spent two restorative years in bed at Colorado Springs. "He came to regard this enforced idleness as one of the most fortunate things that ever happened to him," wrote F. O. Mathiessen. "Looking out at Pike's Peak and meditating on how he wanted to paint, he finally recovered, as he said, from having been a student too long."[24] Later in his convalescence Cheney was joined by the American author H. Phelps Putnam who, ill himself with asthma, sought restoration at the foremost City of Sunshine in the Rocky Mountains.

If a handful of Cragmor's invalids inspired their cohorts by dint of talent, one very wasted consumptive did so by an example of fortitude. Carrie Parsell was only seventeen when in 1914 she was brought to the sanatorium. She spent seven long, discouraging years in bed, a kind of protracted stay-of-execution that would have shattered most ambitions and poisoned normal pleasures. As the weeks and months dragged on and the disease continued to destroy her, Carrie Parsell never uttered a word of complaint. Forster, who treated her through twenty-five hundred days of agony, wrote that "her eyes seemed to hold the only spark of life left to her .... She lay very quietly on her porch with death at her elbow .... She never asked questions as to what the outcome would be, but I am sure she knew the odds were against her. She had a grim little smile that was always ready, and her philosophy seemed to tell her that life was good just as long as it lasted and no matter what it contained." Gradually the tide turned in her favor. She gained weight, lost her fever, and her crippled limbs could once again support her weakened frame. Death had been so close that when she did begin to recover, her case brought new hope and courage to hundreds of others whose bodies were also wracked by tuberculosis. In Forster's opinion, Carrie Parsell loomed as Cragmor's finest example of heroism, a young woman whose outlook typified the kind of spirit that he hoped would become the hallmark of his sanatorium. He carried her name about for years. He told her story to many whining and fretful patients who seemed to need the lesson of an exemplary tale.[25]

Forster was forced to temporarily abandon Carrie Parsell and his Cragmor patients with the outbreak of World War I. When the United States entered the war in the spring of 1917, he was abruptly called to serve in the United States Marine Corps. First ordered to duty in the state of Washington, he was later transferred to San Antonio, then to New Haven, and finally, with the rank of lieutenant colonel, he was placed in charge of an evacuation hospital in France. There he met a young woman from a prominent family of Nantes. The courtship was signally brief, owing both to Forster's broken French and Mademoiselle Liane's unventilated English. On May 1, 1918, the couple were married abroad.

Meanwhile, Cragmor too was affected by the war in Europe. As the conflagration spread its tendrils deeper into the American economy, all hospitals, sanatoriums, and health resorts—both public and private—were alerted to the need to admit indigent patients. For Cragmor this meant swarms of sick people assigned to fill its beds with no thought to their income or earning powers. Quite suddenly, the institution's stockpile of wealthy lungers was drastically reduced, with a corresponding diminution in return for many unhappy investors in Colorado Springs. Many of those who could afford the luxury of a long convalescence preferred to do so at home; the war did much to return scattered consumptives to their families back East.

The real beginning of Cragmor's golden age dates from the end of the war. Soon after the armistice, the sanatorium was again on its way to becoming the nation's most important private cure center for tuberculosis, a feat that could only be accomplished through the resourceful management of its medical superstars, notwithstanding the personal differences that occasionally cropped up between Forster and Webb. Forster, for his part, directed the growth of an ambitious construction era, the end result of which was the founding of a large village colony unlike anything of its kind in the medical world. Webb, in his quiet and sophisticated way, guided the development of a unique educational plan. Between the two of them, Forster and Webb attracted an impressive array of distinguished physicians and nurses to Cragmor. They improved its physical facilities;

they provided superior rehabilitative treatment for tuberculous patients; and they instilled a sense of pride in the youthful lungers that they were in the best cure facility of its kind in the United States, the envy of every hospital from Saranac Lake in New York to the mammoth complex at Fitzsimons in Denver. It was no wonder that by 1924 Cragmor was heralded by the National Tuberculosis Association as "the most desirable sanatorium in the world."[26]

Upon his return from France, Forster recognized that expenses were mounting so rapidly that the only way he could keep Cragmor solvent would be to increase its capacity. Consequently, again he called upon the always dependable Thomas MacLaren and asked him to design a new three-story structure that would occupy a spot thirty feet to the southwest of the existing Main Building, connected to it by a closed corridor. MacLaren came up with an ingenious plan. Estimated to cost $80,000, it assured complete privacy for the occupants of thirty-nine outdoor sleeping porches. Each room in the building required a jog in the wall, and no single porch overlooked the room or porch of its neighbor. Faintly reminiscent of George Edward Barton's building-block concept, the front of each unit would extend several feet beyond the next, thus providing two outside fronts for every patient.[27]

The Cragmor board met and ecstatically endorsed the plan.[28] MacLaren had succeeded again. Actual construction was scheduled to commence in September of 1919, but by October the ground was still unbroken.[29] Early winter storms then moved in, and for reasons undivulged to press or memoir, MacLaren's novel blueprint was permanently scrapped. In its place a less expensive fourth floor was added to the Main Building, topped by another roof garden.[30] Thirty new living quarters, each consisting of a sleeping porch and a private room, divided by a shared bathroom unit, increased the Cragmor's capacity by 50 percent. Moreover, twelve units were added to the administration hall, known henceforth as the Home. The building enterprise of 1920 thus enabled the sanatorium to accommodate a total of 105 patients. It also allowed Forster to pay off a considerable amount of Cragmor's building bonds and to satisfy a number of debts that had accumulated during his absence.[31]

As Cragmor boomed, so did Colorado Springs. Five years earlier only 50,000 tourists had visited the city. Now, in 1920, over 200,000 were expected to flood the community. A critical shortage of housing facilities goaded some local businessmen into planning the construction of three hundred emergency cottages in the downtown area, part of a massive "tent city" project intended to handle the overflow tourists. An architect was hired to design a makeshift colony, but by April that idea too was dropped. "Business judgment," the news media reported, "holds that the expenditure would not be justified under existing conditions."[32]

Forster's next building effort was his most enduring contribution to the Cragmor community. Years earlier at Eudowood he had fashioned a thriving and independent farm colony out of a dreary countryside sanatorium. Removing his bored and melancholy patients from drab, little rooms, he had placed gloves on their hands, straw hats on their heads, and had sent them to plow fields, milk cows, and harvest corn. The curative value of that enterprise was miraculous, claimed Forster, and he ever after maintained that the best tonic for ill health was fresh air, sunshine, supervised manual labor in moderation, and the continuing effort, even by those confined to a state of semiinvalidism, to work for a livelihood. His Eudowood experience was the catalyst behind the birth of Cragmor Village.

"I envision a colony unique in the annals of the medical profession and in the sanatoria world," Forster informed a Colorado Springs reporter, choosing terms familiar to the language of Cragmor's legacy of hyperbole. "In the past tuberculosis patients have often been compelled to surrender all connection with the outside world in order to make a business of living and getting well. At Cragmor it is planned to bring the industry to the patient."[33] Fashioned after the home of the Roycrofters, a society founded by Elbert Hubbard at East Aurora, New York, the extensive cottage colony and industrial center that Forster envisioned for Cragmor would consist of several machine shops; a series of garages; a complex of greenhouse and gardening facilities; printing, illumination, and bookbinding shops; a wagon repair area; pottery, woodcarving, and painting workshops; a dairy farm; and multiple residential units for convalescing lungers and their families. "We have been testing this project on a smaller scale since 1920," claimed Frank M. Houck, the house manager. "Much of the industrial plan must await the passing of the years."[34]

In point of fact, even with the passing of the years the novel guild plan never came to fruition. It died on the planning board, yet another victim of numerous disagreements and a tightening economy. Forster's manufacturing plan was intended to train patients in the work of various professions, partly to pay their expenses at the sanatorium, but largely to provide therapeutic outlets to enhance their recovery. In this respect Forster was years ahead of his time; the big stress on occupational therapy would come much later.

A small portion of Forster's utopian plan was successful—the construction of a model village, consisting in time of nineteen family cottages built along the bluff and out across an extensive tract of land to the south and slightly to the east of the Main Building. By 1924 the Village consisted of eight such structures, thus raising Cragmor's capacity to 113 patients. While more than fifty units of this kind were anticipated, only five additional cottages went up in 1925 and six more were added the following year. Each edifice was a private home with a stucco exterior, tiled bathrooms, stone fireplaces, and inside plumbing. The Village was designed expressly for the benefit of patients or their families, allowing the invalid to remain under a modified sanatorium regime after completing his or her preliminary convalescent period in the sanatorium proper.[35]

The single feature that distinguished the Cragmor cottages from other country bungalows was the presence of a large Solly-MacLaren sleeping porch on the south and southwest side of each structure. Forster called this innovation "the keynote of Cragmor's development. . . . We like our patients and their visitors to become hardened and accustomed to the beneficial effects of good, cold fresh air," he said.[36] Some cottage dwellers had to agree. "It was very bracing," claimed Harriett Cowles of Spokane. "I found it a joy to sleep in the raw in the cold open air."[37] But another porch survivor felt differently: "I was delirious with cold! I nearly froze to death on that beastly porch. But I stayed there, night after night after night, for three long winters. Dr. Forster led me to believe that God had devised the sleeping porch solely for my recovery. So I gritted my chattering

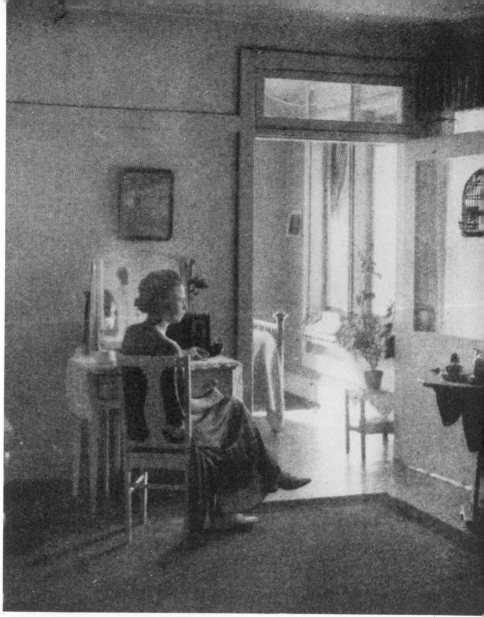

A Laura Gilpin photo, winter 1925

teeth and prayed to Him not to let me die of exposure on His porch before He cured me of consumption."[38]

The Village represented an initial investment of $50,000. It was incorporated in order that an independent board of directors could approve rentals or undertake repairs in the furnished and unfurnished houses without having to consult the more patriarchal Cragmor corporation.[39] However, householders in the convalescent colony secured their food and other supplies by tray service from Cragmor and light, water, telephones, and medical supervision also came from the Main Building. This relieved the institution of the expense of maintaining two separate establishments and allowed for open communication between the sanatorium and its satellite bungalows. Several Village families came with children, so for the first time the sanatorium chasers heard the laughter and chatter of youngsters at play.

Among the first occupants of the new cottages were Ishbel MacLeish, sister of the celebrated poet laureate and dramatist, Archibald MacLeish; Mrs. Audobon Tyler, a renowned artist from Chicago; Ethel Bacharach, playgirl par excellence who advertised her charms as being "free, white, and twenty-one"; Gardiner Hawkins, a graduate of Princeton and future criminal lawyer; Marion W. Sells of Buffalo, whose mother built the first cottage in the new complex for the care of invalids of limited means; and Dr. Brooks D. Good, a tuberculous patient who later became one of Cragmor's most beloved physicians. The Village soon gained a reputation as the preferred place to recuperate. One of its dwellers called it "a swinging retreat on the dusty plain where Prohibition had no place."[40]

A family of two could live in the Village within a budget of two hundred dollars a month. Priority was always extended to married couples; however, several single patients also clamored for a chance to rent a distant and quiet colony villa. The last series of cottages to be built was nestled among newly planted groves of trees, their charm accentuated by a coveted remoteness from the night watchman and curious nurses. Some of Cragmor's most festive parties, gambling bouts, drunken brawls, and discreet affairs took place in those pleasant hamlets of the Village. The cottages were thus the site of many a joyous recovery as well as an occasional grim relapse.[41]

Behind the Village over the hill on the east side of the bluff a remarkable footpath was designed. Dr. Frank M. Houck conceived the pathway plan, then single-handedly surveyed the terrain, leveled mounds of dirt, planted stones, and laid out a delightsome countryside walk as near to a level plane as he could fashion. The pathway, which patients dubbed "Happy Walk," provided Cragmor's inmates with three and one-half miles of strolling pleasure. It completely encircled the bluffs, passing by Coyotes' Den and extending over the uninhabited foothills of the Garden Ranch valley. Houck staked off every fifty feet along the path so that ambulatory consumptives could keep track of the distance they had traveled as part of their open-air treatment.

Houck's popular fresh-air route was known in decorous terms as "the Twilight Sparking Ground," though a less-respectful lunger called it "the High Trail to Passion." "More than one young lady became a victim of a young man's fever on that pathway," complained one employee who had missed all the fun. Yet another recalls two dangers connected with the walkway: "I don't know which creature caused me the most concern out there, my male escort by night or a rattler by day. In either case I had to deal with a snake in the grass."[42]

Much to his sorrow, one elderly gentleman suffered a direct encounter with a rattlesnake on Houck's Happy Walk. Late one afternoon while strolling about a mile from the sanatorium, the old man sat down to rest on a large boulder. He failed to notice the reptile coiled in sleep just behind him and leaned back with his hand resting next to the viper's head. A search party was summoned when he failed to report to dinner. They found him in a state of shock some twenty feet off the trail where he had tumbled down a ravine. He died three days later. The doctors attributed his death to heart failure. For several months after that occurrence, Houck's lovely bucolic trail experienced a marked decline in popularity. The large knoll where the old man met his fate has since been called "Rattlesnake Hill."[43]

Snakebite was only a minor nuisance during the early Roaring Twenties. There was simply too much hard living to do at Cragmor to warrant any lasting concern over countryside venom. The institution's capacity throng of restless lungers thrived on local action and those who deliberately sought it found pleasure in abundance. Forster had long before given his fold a carte blanche for self-governance: "At Cragmor we try not to have any rules. . . . Our patients make their own rules. Individualism is the secret of success in handling tuberculosis."[44]

Most of the patients found reasonably harmless outlets to release their pent-up energies and to combat the ennui of a lengthy bed rest. One such activity was a jovial mock spectacle of unusual events called "Cragmor Rodeo," held annually every

July for nearly ten years. The program was normally staged in an arena roped off directly in front of the Main Building. The 1924 festivity was typical. The first event consisted of a Championship Sputum Cup Folding Contest. "A great deal of rivalry developed during the contest," wrote the associate editor of Cragmor's fortnightly newspaper. "One of the entries sustained a severe fracture of the thumb nail while turning a tight corner." Other stirring events included diving half-naked from an outside window ledge into a bath cot filled with perfumed water; a torrid wheelchair race round Big Circle Drive; high-speed bed baths performed by unblushing nurses on loinclothed patients. The most memorable event of the day was the so-called Roman Race, devilishly described as "patients riding nurses." A large field entered this event. "However," reported one observer, "a number of entries had to be scratched because of the shortage of nurses, several declining to be ridden any longer."[45]

Another activity to ward off boredom was the Cragmor bridge party. Held weekly in the recreation hall, it began as a modest social hour in the fall of 1922, then ultimately expanded into a sophisticated private club, replete with gambling limits, medals, trophies, and spiked refreshments.

On a different evening each week the invalids were invited to Cragmor's full-length films. The first of many first-run silent movies began one October evening in 1924. Spectators came from all over Austins Bluffs to attend the premier show, a film entitled *The Cricket on the Hearth*. Stretchers, wheelchairs, and automobiles lined up in front of the screen on the front lawn. "There was some question," reported the institution's paper, "as to whether it would be possible to see the picture from as high as the fourth floor, but it was found that the height made no difference. In fact, there was one interested spectator who remained on the roof during the entire showing of the film." Most of the patients sat at windows in the Main Building to watch the first of Cragmor's weekly Hollywood specials.[46]

While the world war had required Cragmor to admit a mishmash of the very ill with the least ailing, the cheerless poor with the nouveau riche, hedonistic boozers with reactionary teetotalers, Forster's chief concern was still that of attracting prosperous and well-educated patients. Indeed, one of the institution's abiding distinctions was its large body of celebrated personalities who mixed in with the others. One such illustrious person was the novelist Robert E. McClure, who began *The Dominant Blood* at Cragmor in 1922. Published by Doubleday two years later, the novel was named among the best works of fiction of 1924 and was reviewed by Eva Goldbeck for its "sureness and skill" as a work of "substance and a well-bred air."[47]

Another stellar figure was Robert Reid (1862–1929), the renowned painter and muralist, a partner in Spencer Penrose's Broadmoor Art Academy. While recovering his broken health at Cragmor, Reid did several paintings, some of which later formed a part of permanent collections throughout the country.[48]

The prolific inventor Ira A. Weaver (1871–1965), who founded the largest factory in the world devoted to the manufacture of automotive service equipment, used his leisure time at Cragmor to good advantage. He spent most of the two years of his convalescence inventing the first four-plate brake tester, the Weaver hydraulic press, a car wash pump, and a wheel-alignment tester. In the course of his long life Weaver obtained fifty-eight United States patents; he was once listed as one of the country's most skilled inventors since Edison.[49]

One of the Pikes Peak area's best-known financial wizards began his career in stocks and bonds at Cragmor. Henry Chase Stone from Staten Island was stricken with intestinal tuberculosis the same year that he graduated from Cornell University as president of his class. He arrived at Cragmor on June 26, 1924, and remained at the sanatorium for ten years.[50] During the early stages of his convalescence he took up the art of leather tooling, later directed a private airplane rental at Alexander Field, and eventually became interested in the brokerage business. After his release from Cragmor, Chase Stone worked his way to prominence as one of Colorado Springs most successful financial leaders and midtown builders. He was president of the First National Bank from 1951 until his death in 1966. Today his name is listed with William J. Palmer, Winfield Scott Stratton, and Spencer Penrose as representing the community's most productive, wealthy, and influential citizens.

Cragmor was also an apprenticeship for two accomplished actresses. One was the renowned monologuist, Ruth Draper (1884–1956), whose repertory of some forty sketches in which she portrayed fifty-eight different characters had its beginning in the Women's Cottage on Austins Bluffs. Before making her first national tour as a professional entertainer, Miss Draper polished many of her impersonations before an awed and appreciative audience of fellow convalescents. Using a plain backdrop and only a table and chair, she practiced over and over her remarkable changes with hat and shawl, employing several foreign languages and a wide range of dialects to evoke new character roles, all to the delight of Cragmor's fevered tenants. While still a chaser at Cragmor, she revised parts of the two-hour, two-woman show that she had debuted at Aeolian Hall in London in 1920. Soon after leaving the sanatorium she presented a program that she had first rehearsed before Cragmor's patients in a command performance before King George V and Queen Mary at Windsor Castle.

The second Cragmor thespian of note was Cornelia Skinner, daughter of the famous actor-dean of the American stage, Otis Skinner. A tall, lanky, dark-haired, and only slightly ailing consumptive at twenty years of age, Miss Skinner later informed the world that she had spent the summer of 1922 "vacationing" in Colorado. There was, after all, a strong social stigma attached to the notion of being tubercular. "Vacationing in Colorado" was a common euphemism that many ex-lungers found useful to protect a promising career. Some Cragmorites remember their sudden fright in seeing the dark-haired beauty declaiming in a loud voice from the edge of a precipice high on the bluff, her arms outstretched, reciting Shakespeare to the hills and plains. That fall Cornelia Otis Skinner launched an acting career for herself at Bryn Mawr, where she won the part of Lady Macbeth in the school play. She later went on to Broadway, Hollywood, and the London stage.

Cragmor also had its share of monied kooks. Consider the case of the eccentric patient who paid Fred Russell, the sanatorium driver, three dollars once a month to take him to town to deliver a secret letter to Mrs. Spencer Penrose. Alarmed over his brash impertinence, Mrs. Penrose called the sheriff and had the young swain referred to Brady's Hospital for psychiatric treatment.[51] Or consider the condemned and cynical millionaire poet, Arthur Jeffrey Newman, who decided to face his terminal condition with a sardonic contempt for death and share it with others. He painted many mournful sayings, graffiti, and disease-related posters about the sanatorium grounds and in the Main Building. On the door of the blood bank he inscribed the name Hemorrhage Haven. On the laboratory wall he wrote Pneumothorax Niche. Expectoration Canal greeted lungers in the latrine, while a sign saying Opening of Pleural Cavity announced the first segment of Dr. Houck's pathway back of the bluff. He spent a fortune to place an eight-foot sign atop the craggy heights of Rattlesnake Hill that said Lung Collapse Chasm. Newman also left little rolled-up messages inside napkin holders—cryptic reminders of life's transience and his own nihilistic outlook: "You are sick, I am sick, the world is dying"; and "Do it now; tomorrow you too will be nameless dust." Forster branded this fellow "an enemy of the house." He ordered the signs removed and instructed Newman to desist his sadistic games or forsake the premises. He chose to leave.[52]

Thus Cragmor entered its era of consummate splendor—its cottages and suites catering to the elite, its register reading like the guest list at a Hollywood garden party. On one occasion a fashionable entrepreneur came to the sanatorium from New York. He stayed only five weeks, but when he left he took with him two of Cragmor's maids and one attractive nurse to help him run his Long Island mansion. Forster called it "a vile theft of our most cherished products."[53]

Cragmor's international mélange of patients was well matched by an international set of physicians. These included Charles H. Boissevain, a tall, blond, handsome Dutchman from Amsterdam; Eric Roland Webb, who hailed from the same English town as Gerald B. Webb; and J. Louis Labarerre, a versatile Frenchman whose accomplishments at the piano and the chessboard were exceeded only by his unrivaled expertise on the Byzantine Empire.

The Cragmor was a resort to command respect. Its food was served on nothing less than silver trays in a dining hall that enjoyed a reputation for gastronomic eminence. The table settings always included real china and monogrammed napkins. The regulation dress for entrance into the plush hall was strictly coat and tie. Even tray service for patients confined to bed was maintained under the direction of a professional dietitian. Every room in that splendid asylum was filled. And a lengthy list

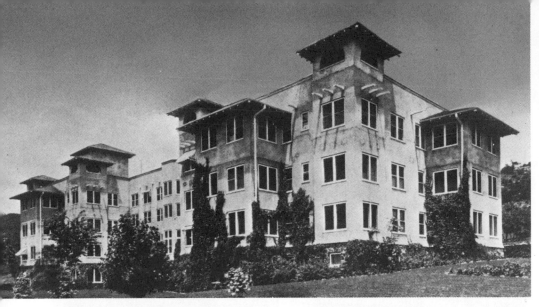

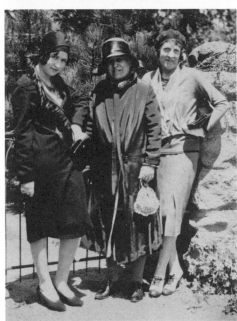

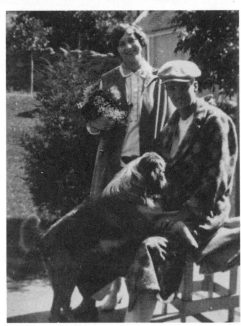

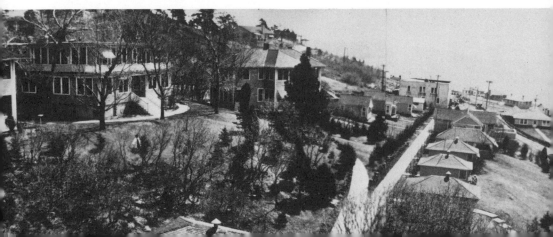

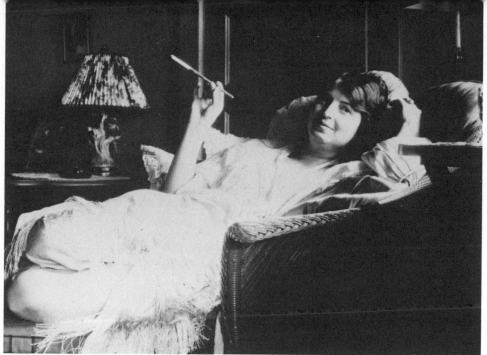

Cragmor's golden age was characterized by the presence of many wealthy and debonair convalescents. The four-story Main Building, the cottages of the Village, the walkways, and the well-groomed lawns, trees, shrubs, and flowers made an ideal environment for patients during the sanatorium's heyday of opulence.

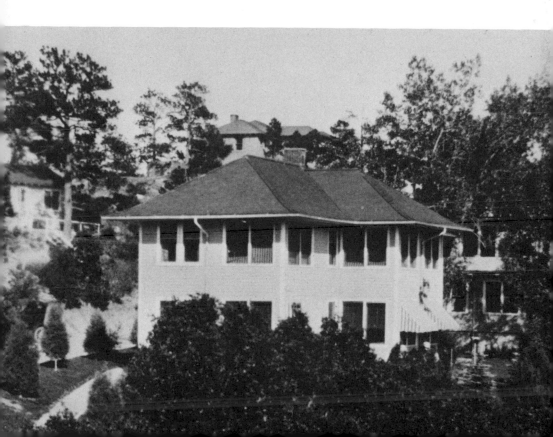

contained the names of lungers waiting impatiently for new openings. The early 1920s signaled the commencement of the institution's golden age of pretense, pomp, and poshness. Cragmor was known as the place where, if you were fortunate enough to be admitted, your convalescence would be such a merry chase that the mere thought of going back home could easily induce a relapse.

Of the more than seven hundred patients who entered and departed Cragmor during its next thirty-six months of regal splendor, the institution's physician-in-chief tried to please them all. He greeted them warmly, granted them free use of the facilities, and asked only that they achieve the maximum contentment permitted by a horizontal life. Boyd St. Clair, one of the editors of Cragmor's fortnightly journal, wrote these words about Forster's positive outlook and unwavering friendliness: "I shall never forget his graciousness, his ability to put me at ease, his light heartedness in the face of my dismal attitude."[54] Forster insisted that the nearly thirty members of his medical staff and the over one hundred employees under his command share his commitment "to create an atmosphere . . . conducive to happiness and cheerfulness" for every inmate.[55]

A few old-timers remained at Cragmor for many years. New patients, as well, tended to prolong their stays beyond the former average of ninety days. Clara Triplett from Mississippi was one such example. She was only twenty years old when she arrived, spent three full years chasing the cure and her man, a dining room waiter, married him, and settled down to live in the community. Many so-called long-term invalids hoped to stay on at Cragmor beyond the time of their scheduled release, and with good reason. The food was superb, the medical care unrivaled, and sanitary conditions were said to be so fine that a wayward germ could die of loneliness. Murray Marcus called Cragmor "the world's choicest place in which to be sick."[56]

Forster attempted to discharge most of the incipient tuberculars within six months. "He practically had to throw me out," claimed one patient. "I left Cragmor with clean lungs and a buoyant heart, but with a knot in my throat as well, knowing that I was departing the home I truly loved."[57] Not all shared her sentiment. One of the shortest and saddest visits was that of Jenefer Hanks from Washington. She had lost two husbands to phthisis and spent nearly three years in bed before entering Cragmor. Covered with lesions and broken in spirit, she left Cragmor on the morning of her twenty-first day at the resort.[58]

But Jenefer Hanks was truly the exception in those days. The emphasis at Cragmor was on good living, right thinking, and long, happy days in the sun. Among the many chasers in 1926 were thirty optimistic students, a score of undespairing housewives, ten ambitious salesmen, forty confident professional people, and a handful of merry youngsters. Also listed as patients were six physicians and one dentist, all of them too disabled to continue their medical practices but willing to spend whatever time was required to recover their health. Once cured, most of them remained at Cragmor as members of its medical staff. Thirty states and seven different countries were represented on Cragmor's roster that year. The youngest patient was five years old, the oldest, fifty. The average age was twenty-seven. Tuberculosis was clearly the disease of young people.

The most popular pastimes among Cragmor's female invalids were bridge and cribbage. The men, for their part, showed a penchant for blackjack and motoring. Concerts, lectures, dramatic skits, movies, and special entertainment continued to flourish. Through the efforts of Rabbi Louis J. Kopald, money was solicited to purchase a Mason and Hamlin grand piano for concerts in the dining hall. The first donor was none other than the Broadmoor's wealthy dowager, Mrs. Charles A. Baldwin, formerly known as Virginia Hobart, the mining heiress from San Francisco. Her philanthropic gesture gave impetus to a rash of donations from other cultural-minded Broadmoorites, and within five months the elegant piano was fully paid for. Rabbi Kopald was furious to hear one sprightly lunger playing ragtime on the prized instrument, so he initiated a second fund-raising campaign to buy an inexpensive upright piano "for such barbaric frivolousness as jazz and the like."[59]

Fine musicians performed at Cragmor. E. Robert Schmitz, recognized as the greatest living interpreter of Bach and modern music, gave a Cragmor recital, as did Margaret Dietrich, a violinist from Leipzig.[60] For three uninterrupted seasons the dining hall featured outstanding cultural events, including one opera (Cademan's *A Witch of Salem*), a concert by the Russian Symphonic Choir, dramatic readings by professional entertainers, and a series of lectures on drama, art, music, history, and phi-losophy. On two evenings a week during the summer of 1925—wedged between the silent movies and the bridge parties—beds and wheelchairs were hoisted up the elevator and pushed into the recreation area so that bedridden patients could attend Cragmor's new "educational convalescence school," the asy-lum's first extension program of formal education. It was spon-sored by a downtown private enterprise called "student corner," directed by Harriett L. Raines. The original faculty consisted of the Australian poet Ernest G. Moll, who offered a short story course; a Spaniard named Felix S. Cobello, who taught French, Spanish, and Italian; and Clara Wilm, who directed a class in German.[61]

The ivy-trimmed walls of Cragmor were a showplace for the region. A luxuriant garden encircled the greenhouse, located at the entrance of the Village, from which fresh vegetables and an abundance of flowers and plants were supplied to the guests. Most of the suites, sleeping porches, and window sills were ar-rayed with home-grown gladiolas, salpiglossis, Oriental pop-pies, hyacinths, narcissi, mums, pansies, tulips, and Queen Anne's lace. For Christmas week, 1927, Mr. Walters, the florist, spun over two thousand feet of evergreen roping to decorate the front halls of the Main Building and the dining hall. Two sum-mers before he had successfully crossed the Pompon and the Show Dahlia to produce a new variety of flower that he called the "Cragmor." Its bright yellow center, surrounded by glowing ruby-red petals, could be seen for several summers thereafter on the window ledges and rooftop of the Main Building, only to be replaced each September by asters and carnations. The Cragmor greenhouse was one of the largest and most productive floral gardens in the Pikes Peak region.

Clustered about the sanatorium grounds were thirty group-ings of lilac bushes. According to one practicing ornithologist, sixty species of birds flocked to Cragmor's fields and protective trees every year.[62] "Cragmor was a paradise," reported Maude Boulton, who spent three years of her life confined to a bed in the Women's Cottage. "There was no other place on earth I would have rather been."[63] Boyd St. Clair wrote that the sanato-rium that first greeted him in the early spring of 1923 was "dull grey, drab, penitentiary-like," but that within only two years it had become "a haven of beauty."[64]

A minibuilding boom took place between the spring of 1924 and midsummer of 1927, including the construction of The Little Shop, a combination drug and grocery store on the third floor of the Main Building, where patients could buy magazines, cigarettes, candy, cosmetics, and stationery.[65] At the same time a barber shop and a beauty salon were built on the ground floor, each serviced by professional haircutters and beauticians from the Springs. Major M. Fennell, who cut hair at Cragmor until 1934, recalls charging twenty–five cents per haircut, twice that amount for a room call, and five dollars to shave a dead person.[66]

Attesting to Cragmor's spirited independence and resourcefulness was the short-lived effort during the mid-1920s to mint an institutional brass token in various denominations. The coins never entirely replaced paper or silver currency, of course, but they enjoyed frequent use in The Little Shop and at the Village gambling tables. Today they are esteemed as a rare and sought–after item of historical curiosity.[67]

Another addition was a small post office near the Main Building's front entrance. It remained in operation for nearly ten years. Cragmor boasted an amazing airmail service record. In July of 1924, for instance, a letter took only thirty hours for delivery from New York City. "Surely the American Postal Department has commenced an epoch in rapid transcontinental mail delivery," falsely prophesied the editor of *Ninety-Eight-Six*.[68]

Still another renovation was the erection in the recreation hall of two walls of bookshelves to facilitate moving Cragmor's modest library from the Home, where it was first established in 1924, into the Main Building in 1926. Cragmor's first library consisted of 811 volumes (February 1925); that count increased to 1,170 by September of 1926. A library catalog was placed in every room. Patients were permitted to keep books for one month. Although half of the books on loan were never returned, the librarian did not institute a policy of fines. Gerald Webb encouraged his patients to keep the books that they liked. In reality, the only appropriation that bothered Cragmor's staff was the all–too–frequent removal of bed linen and silverware, a common practice among souvenir–minded invalids.

Other refurbishings extended to the grounds surrounding the sanatorium. The straight cement walkway that linked the Main Building with the employee's dormitory was formerly named the Rialto but known after 1925 as the Broadway. It was provided with a sheltered archway of trees and vine arbors. Fifteen residences spanned both sides of the Broadway, including Solly's original cabin, now expanded in size from three small rooms to six ample suites and a sun porch. One annoyed patient called this area "Stentorian Lane," owing to the raucous sound that periodically emanated from nine radios, five victrolas, seven dogs, two cats, and one monkey housed in the vicinity. Indeed, noise was the major cause for complaints at Cragmor, be it from animal, bird, or humankind. Invalids at rest were frequently jarred when pairs of juggernauting, white-clad busboys raced their trays on flat and rhomboid wheels down the busy walkway. Forster scolded his patients repeatedly about "the unearthly racket" at Cragmor. In one memorandum circulated in July of 1925 he objected to slamming doors, throwing furniture about, thumping on the floor with high-heeled shoes, playing phonographs, clashing gears, beeping horns, and noisy late-night debauchers. Yet still he eschewed the imposition of stern measures: "It is our constant hope that by avoiding rigid rules we may . . . create a spirit of cheerfulness."[69]

The sanatorium's favorite stone idol donned the front entrance to the Main Building: a handsome horserack. For many years it represented the institution's proud gateway for equestrian visitors. When Forster discovered that two female patients who had been assigned to a strict rest regimen were sharing horseback rides with a debonair young man from town, he promptly ordered all riding stopped. "It is not the object of the sanatorium to make a trained athlete of the patient," he scolded.

A clock golf green with several lanes leading off into tree-lined botanical gardens was ready for use by July of 1924. The green's opening coincided with an outdoor wedding between Edith Talbot and Mack McCoy, two among the many patients who discovered love among the bacilli. Their nuptials were one of the resort's most festive occasions, inspiring the florist to drape palms, ferns, and peonies in great profusion about the pi-azzas, lanes, and arbors.

Sadly, most of the sanatorium's elaborate garden work was wiped out by a major storm one Saturday morning in August of that year. Heavy rain, hail, and high winds lashed the area with such intensity that the new foundation for the Norris-MacLeish cottage, recently poured, washed down the side of the bluff. Sidewalks too were ripped out, trees uprooted, and the one-month-old botanical gardens and golf green were left in total shambles. It took over two years to restore the broken shrub-bery and mud-strewn trails to their former shape, but the golf green and exquisite gardens were never replaced.

The major construction project of the period was a $30,000 twenty-seven-room, two–storied addition located south of the Main Building. The new building, completed in July of 1927, was designed by Otto B. Engleking. It followed architectural lines similar to those of Thomas MacLaren's Main Building, in-cluding large sleeping porches connected to every room. The unit's only deficiency seemed to be its lack of a suitable name. No one could agree on what to call it. The Cragmor newspaper ran a name contest, patients debated the propriety of one name over another, and doctors and nurses argued the issue. For three months or so the greatest problem at Cragmor seemed to be finding a proper name for the new building. Some opted for "Ed-win Solly Hall," to better perpetuate the name of Cragmor's founder; others preferred "Forster Hall," to honor the living di-rector. Still others insisted on such names as "Windswept Hall" ("because there is not a breeze that blows that does not find its way through its porches and windows"); "Questover Hall" ("be-cause here ends the quest we have all been making"); even "Rom-garc Dormitory" (Cragmor spelled backwards). One young man suggested "South Hall," but the editor of *Ninety-Eight-Six* promptly rejected such a puerile title because "it showed no imagination and was much too obvious." So for the next twen-ty–five years the nameless structure was simply called "the New Building."[70]

Cragmor was so crowded between 1925 and 1928 that new patients could only be admitted on a reservation basis. At one time Laurence L. Cragin, the business manager, announced that the reservation list was filled ten months in advance. There was talk of massive expansion. Forster hoped to cover 950 undeveloped acres with additional cottages plus construct a fifty–room replica of the Main Building just to the north of the sanatorium. However, these lavish plans never materialized. Cragmor was already so large and active a resort that its medical personnel found it an exhausting task to fulfill the needs of 185 patients, as well as those of the families residing in the Village.

The sanatorium proper now covered 140 acres on land valued at $14,254. Its six major buildings, eight cabins, laundry, garage, employees' dormitory, greenhouse, and horse stable were valued at $578,202. Cragmor Village covered another 550 acres and consisted of nineteen homes valued at $105,000. These rented for between $75 and $125 per month. In 1926 the weekly rental for a cabin was $25–35, for the cottage apartments $30–40, and for a private bath accommodation in the Main Building, $50–60. By the middle of 1927 Cragmor's lunger population reached a new all–time capacity load of 235 individuals, counting those who were chasing the cure in the Village.[71] The institution was then recognized as the largest privately operated sanatorium in the world.[72] The medical community prized Cragmor for two reasons: one, because Forster managed its operation without an endowment; and two, because it combined a unique development of institutional care with residential convalescence.[73]

The sanatorium was especially celebrated for its rooftop sun cure healing methods. Indeed, heliotherapy, or sun treatment, gave the institution its main call to fame from 1914 through the late 1930s. In the winter, heliotherapy was administered daily between ten in the morning and four in the afternoon, while in the summer it was given before eleven in the morning and after three in the afternoon. It consisted of mat-prone, cot-reclining, bed-sprawled sunbaths in loincloth attire or full nudity amidst the inspiring potted greenery on the Main Building's roof garden. In 1926 special booths were erected to insure a relative degree of privacy, but even those wind-blown partitions proved inefficient as soon as Chase Stone began renting private planes at Alexander Field, piloted by expert aviators who gladly accommodated their clients' whims, especially if after a handsome tip they were directed to dip low over Cragmor's rooftop.[74]

The literature lauding the benefits and techniques of helio-

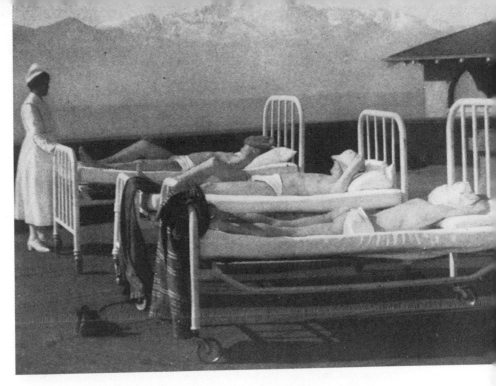

therapy at Cragmor has a long and curious history, amply recorded in the pages of *Ninety-Eight-Six*.[75] Sunbathing alone accounted for the attraction of more than half of the sanatorium's inmates. They came with pallid, emaciated bodies, sought a daily dosage of salubrious rays while lying prostrate for many hours under the tanning glow of Colorado's sun, only to emerge many months or even years later in plumpness and health, their darkened skins cracked and weathered after a long tenure of chasing in the sun. The "Solar Knights," as they were dubbed, represented Cragmor's most devoted practitioners of immobilized insolation.

Naturally those who failed to heed the doctors' instructions often sustained considerable damage from excessive sun exposure. One woman had to be transferred to Glockner to be treated for sunstroke. It would be interesting to study how many among Cragmor's overripe sun worshipers may have contracted skin cancer in later years. According to one early medical account, the state of Colorado had a bad name as a resort area for chasing the cure because too many patients soaked up too much sun, sustained high temperatures, and died.[76] Nevertheless, it was overexertion, not excess sunlight, that accounted for most of the deaths at Cragmor. Dr. Charles E. Sevier was the sanatorium's able supervisor for sun therapy, and he carefully monitored every patient's solar activity on the roof, keeping excess exposure to a minimum.[77]

Cragmorites discovered that their sundeck stint served as a capital therapeutic release from the social whirl of the evening before. Solar rest hours were a good time to "sleep it off." Others conceded that the rooftop was also a dangerous "garden of solar foreplay." They argued that people with tuberculosis were already more highly sexed than normal people because they constantly ran a low fever, and placing them together for hours at a time on "Nudity Flats," as the roof garden was affectionately called, clad only in a flimsy towel or loincloth coverlet, tended to excite their natural inclinations to engage in promiscuous activities, especially when Dr. Sevier was not present. Several of Cragmor's employees, obliged to heed strict rules of segregation and moral conduct in their dormitory units, envied the patients their permissive solar merriment. It was commonly believed that ambulatory consumptives had all the fun at Cragmor: "Dark golden tans hide perfidious plans," ran the aphorism.[78]

The extensive attention given to Cragmor's sun cure led to the invention of Frank Verba's wondrous Solar Therapeutic Laryngoscope, a curious instrument that employed metallic mirrors to hurl heat and sunlight down a patient's throat in the treatment of tuberculous laryngitis. The sanatorium gained international acclaim throughout the medical world for its use of Verba's apparatus. Several professional papers lauding its effectiveness prompted a goodly number of tuberculars with throat disease to flock to the sun resort on Austins Bluffs.

Cragmor's fame and good works also spilled over into the city. When Forster's scheme for building a complex industrial community failed to materialize, the sanatorium turned its attention to a curative workshop downtown. The midtown facility opened on June 1, 1926. Called "Half-Way House," the satellite enterprise was intended to provide health-seekers with occupational therapy on a small scale. Two Cragmorites directed the project in partnership with two women from the Broadmoor area and a professional occupational therapist. Others volunteered to conduct classes and within a short time the new rehabilitation center functioned on a daily schedule. During its first three months of operation, approximately 255 free lessons were offered in such crafts as weaving, basketry, leather and beadwork, sewing, light carpentry, painting and designing, pyralin work, hooked and braided rugs, chair caning, and toy making.

Many convalescents gravitated to the workshops of Half-Way House and in due course it opened its doors to nontuberculars as well, providing occupational and social services for diseased, handicapped, disabled, and addicted citizens of the community. By the fall of 1928 there were 225 patients enrolled in the handicraft classes. Cragmor patients unable to travel to town could secure lessons at the sanatorium for a dollar an hour. In two years the shop gave 5,940 lessons and returned nearly $4,000 in commissions to patients whose work was sold. This profitable business venture became one of the sanatorium's most successful offerings to the community, until it was exceeded in popularity and profits by Navajo beadwork during a later period.[79]

Another source of pride for the Cragmor was the publication of *Ninety-Eight-Six*, so named to reflect the ideal temperature to which its readers were striving. Laura Gilpin praised the sophisticated fortnightly journal as "an example of excellent design and craftsmanship in printing. . . . It is edited so skillfully," she wrote, "that aside from the interest of the contents the presentation of the whole is the best possible advertisement for the institution it represents."[80] The *Colorado Springs Gazette* called it "the most elaborate and artistic publication of the Pikes Peak region."[81]

The founders and editors of *Ninety-Eight-Six* had undisguised literary pretensions. When the publication first appeared in 1917, it was a mere single-sheet gossip weekly, but soon thereafter it evolved into a mimeographed circular of bedside wit and medical tidbits and finally as a full-fledged printed magazine with an aim to balance topical news with outside cultural contributions. During its first three years of publication more than fifty professional writers contributed to its pages, including such luminaries as Stuart P. Sherman, the first editor of the *New York Herald Tribune* literary section, whose son was a patient at Cragmor; Schuyler Ashley, who wrote most of his celebrated short stories while confined to bed; Joseph Carr, the New York poet and artist; Leroy Placet, the former editor of *Little Literary Re-*

view, then in charge of a New York drama group; and H. K. Ellingson, whom Walter Winchell called "a writer of the most interesting and most quoted book reviews in the Rocky Mountain region."[82]

The editors of *Ninety-Eight-Six* tried to make its pages as cosmopolitan as possible and give the patients and doctors free rein for their ideas and effusions. Gerald Webb published several exquisite profiles on tuberculous celebrities, as well as a series of articles on heliotherapy. Forster wrote a regular column in response to questions from patients whose curiosity ranged from the dangers of contamination through necking ("Try it and see," he replied) to problems underlying a delicate pneumothorax operation. And the patients themselves submitted poems, essays, short stories, quips, and homespun sketches. Surprisingly, sentimental gush and rampant self-pity—exhortations to be of stout heart and to fight the good fight—were as rare in *Ninety-Eight-Six* as they were lamentably regular in numerous institutional organs from other sanatoriums.

At times the journal provided a positive and culturally edifying outlet for serious literary aspirations. Schuyler Ashley's reviews on new books (e.g., Ernest Hemingway's *The Sun Also Rises*) and his informative essay entitled "Contemporary American Writers" launched his career as a full-time writer.[83] Equally impressive were occasional poems that found their way out of *Ninety-Eight-Six* and into national anthologies.[84]

Not all of the magazine's contributions were top caliber, of course. There was the usual potpourri of unpolished tales, prissy gossip, and nauseous poems, some so banal that a relapse would have been preferred to a re-reading. From time to time a reviewer's indignant personal evaluation of a new work would cloud objective perception, as might be concluded from the following comment by Charles Ryder about a new novel: "It's too long, too egregious, makes too little concession to its public, and is . . . too obscure to bother about." The book in question was James Joyce's *Ulysses*. In some instances the writing for *Ninety-Eight-Six* was downright atrocious. As the journal rose in esteem with materials submitted by accomplished writers, so too it degenerated several notches by running syrupy little verses and vaporous sketches written by Cragmor's bedridden neophytes of the fourth estate. Nevertheless, despite its breezy jokes and institutional gabble, *Ninety-Eight-Six* was counted among the most prestigious of America's twenty-seven major sanatorium magazines.[85]

Occasional research projects taken up by the Cragmor's fledgling scholars were also published in *Ninety-Eight-Six*. Between December of 1924 and July of 1929, for instance, there was a widespread interest in ornithology at the sanatorium. And what better way to spend one's convalescent hours of the horizontal cure than by observing birds and their fascinating habits? With field glasses and guidebook in hand, many of Cragmor's patients spent countless hours at their windows, on the porches and the roof, strolling across the open fields or along Dr. Frank Houck's secluded pathway, to observe the more than sixty different species of birds that inhabited or visited the area.

The first person to compile extensive findings was Myrtle K. Low from Chattanooga, a graduate of the University of Chicago, and a devoted bird lover. She was a patient at Cragmor from September 1926 through most of 1928. Known as the sanatorium's Bird Lady, Mrs. Low often missed her meals or got herself lost in the hills in pursuit of avian residents. Her interest in birds was so contagious that at one time she had as many as fifty-two invalids addicted to bird watching. "It consumed my life," reported one Cragmorite, "At Mrs. Low's behest, I bought a pair of binoculars, a copy of the *Auk*, and logged in over nine hundred hours studying bird life. Cragmor was then a paradise of small shrubs. Birds were everywhere. The gardener had built many large tree trays for feeding them, and my own pockets were always filled with bread crumbs, suet or hemp seeds to lure them to my side. . . . My notebook contained two hundred pages of handwritten notes on just the common finches, sparrows, and chickadees."[86]

Colorado ranked third among the states in number of recorded birds, with 425 different species and subspecies.[87] A local birdwatcher claimed that one-fourth could be seen from any cottage bedside on Austins Bluffs. Myrtle Low observed many of them on her daily patrols, seeking a quiet retreat with her feathered friends over the hill behind the sanatorium, noting the nesting and living habits of such species as chickadees, nuthatches, woodpeckers, creepers, grosbeaks, towhees, and waxwings. In July of 1927, when she saw two rare visitors on

Cragmor's grounds—a mockingbird and a white robin—she ecstatically ran to the dining hall and announced that the year 1927 would go down in ornithological annals as *annus mirabilis.* Her well-fed bird devotees all stood and cheered.[88]

Myrtle Low's aviary gauntlet was picked up in 1929 by Clinton G. Abbott, who carefully observed the comings and goings of both winter and summer birds at Cragmor. Abbott was much more than an impassioned birdwatcher; his amateur curiosity evolved into the making of a full-time ornithological profession. He lacked only Mrs. Low's intrepid mobility. Owing to a condition that required absolute bed rest, Abbott made all of his observations from a bedside screen in a small wooden cabin near the Broadway Walk. He trained other patients and nurses to respect his communion time with the birds; he was never to be disturbed whenever a large peacock feather flag was seen flapping in the breeze over the front door of his cabin.[89]

While some Cragmorites found delight in winged songsters, others became enraptured by the making, marketing, or guzzling of forbidden firewater. The Eighteenth Amendment meant nothing to Cragmor's avid booze peddlers, and for two or three gentlemen bootlegging became more a livelihood than a clandestine hobby. Just over the hill to the south was the community of Papetown, a lively Italian-American neighborhood where low quality bogus whiskey could be bought and sold with the utmost contempt for the Volstead Act.[90] Alcohol of higher quality could be purchased for the right price at Cragmor. In fact, one of the sanatorium's folk heroes of the Prohibition Era was a man whose professional reputation rested on the illegal transport of intoxicating beverages. His name was Harry Voyles, a flamboyant and mercenary member of Chicago's notorious Purple Gang, who first made a name for himself regulating petty rackets in Chicago saloons. He was primed for larger stakes in interstate liquor commerce, and eventually found his way into the western bootlegging market. He was conveniently stricken with tuberculosis at a time when many of his hapless gangland buddies fell victim to mob reprisals and police bullets, so his rest cure at Cragmor provided Voyles a welcome reprieve from big city violence. It was believed that Voyles's private aircraft stationed at Alexander Field, just down the road from Cragmor, accounted for many clandestine deliveries of the best in bottled rum and whiskey. His interests spread as far south as Pueblo and as near at home as the nightspots in Papetown, but he discreetly kept his prohibition booze out of the reach of the "commoners" at Cragmor. Voyles was notoriously a private man and his business concerns in Colorado still remain a tightly guarded secret.[91]

Birds, flowers, pathways, concerts, journals, books, booze, minted coins, and spacious buildings all attested to the delights of Forster's thriving sanctuary. Cragmor was to TB sanatoriums what Palm Beach was to pleasure resorts; it was a marvel in its time. From the first day of its operation over twenty years before, the sanatorium had grown erratically, often with long leaps and short jerks, some false starts, much backsliding, large heavy thumps, and freewheeling forward spins, skirting dreams of utopian preeminence, falling just short of majesty, but traveling upward on the high road of sanatorium dukedom. At the pinnacle of his own success as the patriarch of this remarkable country health resort, Alexius M. Forster could look back on past accomplishments with a true sense of pride. He had known and enjoyed the good things of life at Cragmor; his sanatorium had the heritage of an aristocratic past. In the womb of an uncertain future, Forster had no thought that the smugness and complacency of the late twenties would very soon shift into the incubus of a sorry decline. Were he as privileged to discern the events of the troubled thirties and dreadful forties as well as he could rejoice over the past, Forster's serenity at age forty-seven would have vanished like the sweet distant song of Cragmor's evanescent meadowlark. Until its bankruptcy and ultimate liquidation forty-five years later, Cragmor would tread a long, slow trail of moral, financial, and physical deterioration.

FIVE

Tarnish and Dissolution

*Cragmor will collapse under
the sheer weight of its own
inherent and incurable infamy.*
Robert W. Sloan

In the course of only two years, Colorado Springs's population jumped from 36,728 to just over 45,000 (1926–28). It was a thoroughly modern town, with evidence of a checkered growth to the north as far out as the vine-covered walls of the Cragmor Sanatorium. From the cottage porches of Forster's debonair resort, consumptives could hear the strains of dance music wafting up from Papetown or the sounds of an orchestra and laughter from the new ballroom on the edge of Alexander Field. Though Prohibition still prevailed, the difference between a cheerful and a fretful patient was often measured by a call down the road and a late-night run into Papetown to procure a bottle of moonshine from some nameless bootlegger's truckload of high-priced oblations.

Until the summer of 1929, Cragmor was a happy, carefree habitation jammed with jaunty lungers and their party-minded visitors. Marshall Sprague recounts how a friend, returning from Denver at three in the morning "when the rest of Colorado Springs was dark as the inside of a cow," looked up to see Cragmor blazing "with light like an ocean liner on cruise—all four floors of it."[1] By day the sanatorium glistened with the elegance of a courtly manor. Old "Dad" White, who had served as its caretaker since 1920, cleared the daily rubbish, mowed the lawns, and trimmed the hedges with such fastidious pains as to transform Cragmor into a tended estate. "To picture the rough plain on which it was built," wrote Boyd St. Clair, "and then to picture the green grass, and trees, and flowers, one is awed by the tremendous amount of work that it has involved. . . . Without doubt, the Sanatorium is one of the most beautiful in the country."[2]

On the surface, activities bubbled much the same as they had before. Few problems plagued the sanatorium in 1928; it remained crowded, smug, and prosperous. Noise was still its cardinal nuisance. The bedridden, or "down-patients," complained about the footloose, or "up-patients," gossiping in the hallways or shouting from atop Cragmor's sun roof to their knicker-clad pals playing croquet on the lawn below. Forster often turned to his column in the institution's newspaper to scold ambulatory inmates about door banging, radio disturbance, and general raucous behavior. One intransigent young man was cured of his irksome habit of singing late at night when twelve self-appointed vigilantes of the common peace entered his room, wrapped him up in a sheet, and carried him out to the front lawn, where they tossed him up and down in a blanket. Thereafter the sanatorium enjoyed many peaceful evenings. No one dared incur the wrath of the "Dreadful Silencers" and their fearsome blanketing.[3]

Movies could still be previewed at Cragmor long before they played at the Broadmoor or in downtown movie houses. In August of 1928 Colorado Springs obtained its first "talkies," an event that inspired several Cragmorites to campaign hard for the purchase of a sound projector. The editors of Ninety-Eight-Six issued a public call for donations and it was not long before the sanatorium's silent film era drew to a close. With the inauguration of weekly Hollywood "talkies," Cragmor was a hive of activity and excitement.

The local bridge scene also changed. Displeased with the casual structure of its open-door policy, the ladies of Cragmor's weekly bridge club formalized their proceedings by electing officers, drafting rules, requiring bimonthly dues, serving sumptuous refreshments, offering high-score prizes, and rotating hostess assignments. Beginning in mid-June of 1930 a twenty-five cent charge was assessed to each player participating in the Thursday evening bridge tournament. Latecomers were fined, newcomers required a formal induction, and delay-of-play tactics resulted in point demerits. "This police action and elitist trend," exclaimed one disgruntled member, "will kill all interest in the game."[4] Her words were prophetic. The highfalutin Cragmor bridge club disbanded in May of 1931 in the wake of an outbreak of angry quarrels among its participants.

Cragmor's other social diversions soon began to wane. Vaudeville revues replaced formal recitals, educational convalescence classes gave way to minstrel shows, and the grand piano had to be dusted more often than it was played. Until the fall of 1929, however, Cragmor was still known as the place to go north of town for the best in classical concerts. Bimonthly programs featured voice and instrumental groups, with occasional solo performances. The last regular recital of the famed "Dining Room Series" took place on September 30, 1929. Thereafter the only public programs were infrequent employee shows held on special occasions, such as the Fourth of July or Easter.[5]

One revue called the "Cragmor Frolics" played every January for three consecutive years (1928–30), but the final production was interrupted when one of the lead performers suffered a hemorrhage and had to be rushed to the infirmary. Owing to that grim incident, the doctors decided that any form of stirring music, tumbling or juggling acts, dancing, or stage shows tended "to quicken the pulse and slow up the cure."[6] They thereby recommended a curtailment of all future "Cragmor Frolics." Forster prohibited "any type of physical exertion," a sweeping edict that not only cancelled many popular handicraft classes sponsored by the downtown Half-Way House but also put a crimp in the educational classes conducted by professors from Colorado College.[7] In their place the doctors organized sedate garden parties, such as the refined fête of July 4, 1930, at which over one hundred patients dressed in pajama ensembles gathered on the front lawn in wheelchairs, ambulance carts, and deck chairs to play innocuous games of chance and sing patriotic songs in unison. One Cragmorite claimed that it took only two of these parties to disprove Cragmor's worldwide reputation as the favorite orgy center of all Western Hemisphere sanatoriums.[8]

As the twenties gradually faded away, genteel lawn picnics became the typical social affairs of Cragmor. "Where have all the parties gone?" queried one baffled ex-patient returning for a visit. "The liquor? the women? the poker games?" He was told that gum-chewing was now the rage and if he wished to indulge his appetities in an authorized sport, he could bend over to untie and tie up his shoelace.[9] Forster's rigid proclamation restricting group activities did not apply to serene picnics, weekly movies, and the ill-fated bridge night, but everything else had to go. "It was a surprising reversal of the doctor's laissez-faire attitude," complained one employee. "From one day to the next the San suddenly shifted from no rules whatever to a strict and uncompromising discipline."[10] The abrupt drying up of many social, cultural, and educational offerings annoyed several old-timers. "Is this a T.B. San or a morgue?" asked one inmate.[11] This echoed an earlier complaint: "The outstanding fault of Cragmor is the lack of social life; the complete absence of a spirit of camaraderie. . . . This stressing of privacy has had a deadening effect."[12] Some individuals felt so betrayed by the ban and the glacial attitude adopted by Cragmor's management that they deserted the establishment for other more active resorts. As new patients replaced them, it was apparent that incipient tuberculars were becoming more rare. Instead, the management was now intent on admitting more advanced cases. By the mid-thirties this policy gave rise to a new perspective. Mental buoyancy and recreation—the themes of Forster's original creed—were replaced by Cragmor's sole concern and raison d'être: disease. As bedridden invalids steadily grew and tray service to the chronically ill increased, the dapper, party-prone playmates of the asylum's sportive past began to dissipate. Conviviality was rapidly limited to a decorous tête-à-tête on the sun deck or a submissive hello on the Broadway Walk. Even Dr. Houck's handsome trail, once the most interesting outdoor attraction at Cragmor, fell into disuse. Now very few patients were even strong enough to follow the scenic pathway, and the few who were did not care to.

Complaints soared and the general morale plummeted. "I have tried to trace the origin of Cragmor's anti-social attitude," wrote one perplexed invalid, who had been vexed because no one spoke to her, "and I see a pertinent significance in the astounding fact that this sanatorium, accommodating over one hundred people, has no salon—no place for people to come together for the exchange of ideas and nonsense." She further objected that teatime was never mentioned at Cragmor. "I broached the idea of having one to a nurse, and she looked incredulous—'Why, my dear, that isn't done here.'"[13]

And there were other distressing incidents. A rash of dog poisoning destroyed most of the pets that once frolicked along the Broadway path. The culprits were never found, but vigilantes patrolled the grounds with blood in their eyes. Nor were the burglars apprehended who accounted for an outbreak of thievery at the sanatorium during the summer and fall of 1929. Money, purses, watches, jewelry, and personal effects—including one woman's autographed portrait of Theodore Roosevelt and a gentleman's mounted insect collection—disappeared from twelve suites, two cabins, and four cottages over a three-month spread of time. The police were baffled; they could uncover no clue of any kind. As no evidence of forced entry was found, many patients claimed that the crimes were perpetrated from the inside. Thus, as more belongings disappeared, suspicions mounted, tempers flared, and the gentle relaxed air for which Cragmor had been noted was replaced by tension.[14] Utopia was in trouble.

Two years before, Forster had warned all "unhappy, disgruntled and self-centered patients" to improve their attitude or get out. "Adaptability is needed in every other relation with life," he said, "and if the patient can not appreciate the fact that it is essential here, then he is certainly better off elsewhere."[15] By 1930 the time was ripe for expulsion. Indeed, as new infractions occurred and as Forster's new rules demanding silence and inactivity were summarily ignored, house evictions increased. For the first time since Solly had been obliged to expel a pair of troublemakers the year that Cragmor opened, patients were again discharged for misconduct. Nor would this be the last time. In later years, under George Dwire's supervision, many behavior problems would have to be resolved by the only effective mechanism of the management's strong will: banishment.

While unsettling problems festered among the sanatorium's bemused and dismayed guests, the once-spirited magazine known as *Ninety-Eight-Six* also encountered hard times. One imbroglio occurred when an irate female reader launched a fervent assault on the journal's "immoral and suggestive indignities." She objected to its "display of pornographic ravings . . .

the sick spewings of mud spattered over our fair pages." Others defended "the frisky fiction" and "sparkling trimmings" of Cragmor's lively organ. If in fact the little publication revealed a penchant for ribaldry, it did so in a very subdued and subtle way. It contains nothing capable of raising an eyebrow today. Yet in 1929 adverse criticism troubled its editors to such a degree that they gave serious thought to terminating the journal's existence.[16]

The pornographic fracas died down in time but it left a residue of petty resentments and divided readership. Once committed to the thankless task of editing a fortnightly literary magazine with an ardor worthy of numerous journalistic citations, the editors of *Ninety-Eight-Six* now found it necessary to agitate for subscriptions, to combat apathy, and to wrestle with rising costs of printing in the early months of the Depression. It is not surprising, therefore, that with the distribution of the February 25, 1932, issue, following another outburst of objections over content and the journal's moral stance, the last of its beleaguered editors packed his typewriter, locked the office door, and resigned his post. For seven and a half years, *Ninety-Eight-Six* had enjoyed continuous publication, but the three villains of the news media—financial hardship, public indifference, and unwarranted censorship—combined in the end to silence its pages.

The stock market crash of October 1929 dealt a severe blow to Cragmor's declining clientele of prosperous lungers. Modest fortunes, gained only a few months earlier, were abruptly lost in the general collapse of industrial, oil, rail, and other stocks. While no collective hysteria was manifested at the sanatorium, several individuals reacted badly. One elderly patient returned to his mercantile business in the East, found it in shambles, and shot himself. Another lunger who had lost his investments and could no longer support his family, died in Palmer Park of a self-inflicted gunshot wound, hoping thereby to leave his wife a sizeable insurance payoff.[17] In 1934 one of the consultants went crazy; he too had lost considerable money in stocks and had to be forcibly removed from Cragmor and transferred to Brady's Hospital for psychiatric care. Others who had lost their life's earnings merely packed up their remaining goods and returned with active bacilli to their homes. The advent of the Great De-

pression marked an end to Cragmor's aristocratic past and signaled the beginning of a bourgeois population, which as time
advanced became more and more frayed about the edges.

By February of 1930 all of the cabins, except for the Solly,
were deserted. Several Cragmor Village homes were also va-
cated and attempts were made to rent them out during hard
times for a nominal fee. There was a major turnover in the staff.
The capable dietitian, Helene Barbee, who had been on the payroll since July of 1919, left the sanatorium to secure a graduate
degree at Johns Hopkins. Several replacements for her position
came and went over the years, few working out to great satisfaction. Jim Webb, Cragmor's head waiter, an ex-miner and former valet for an English lord, ended his life one afternoon over
a case of unrequited love by consuming a full bottle of cyanide
in the restroom of the Chief Theater.[18] His replacement, Theo
Gildson, came to Cragmor from San Francisco's plush Bohemian
Club, trailing letters and a resplendent folio attesting to his reputation as one of California's finest chefs. For a few years he
struggled to maintain the smug dignity of the sanatorium's
dining hall, introducing such innovations as printed menus,
guest lists, and name cards, but the formal trappings seemed all
too anachronistic in an era of broken sophistication, when patients shuffled in to eat wearing bedroom slippers and robes
rather than coats, ties, and carnations.

Cragmorites seemed happiest when left alone to bask in the
sun or to fill their ailing lungs with the crisp mountain air of a
Colorado night. Forster continued to urge his patients to sleep
in isolation on their porches in all seasons. When the sharp, dry
winds of January battered the asylum, he reminded the frozen
denizens of the Solly school-of-the-fresh-air-cure to remain in
their refrigeration units in zero temperatures: "The tonic effect
of cold weather is most beneficial," he wrote. Yet within six
weeks of that reassuring pronouncement *Ninety-Eight-Six* reported that colds, flu, and bronchitis were running wild about
the sanatorium.[19]

However, the fear of contracting pneumonia never deterred
Cragmor's stalwart porch fanatics. They threw back the sashes,
opened all doors and windows, and invited the biting cold
winds to sweep through their rooms, halls, passageways, and
into the diseased filaments of their lungs. Ironically, the only re-

ported tragedy to ensue from the fresh-air fetish was the loss of Forster's own child. He had insisted on leaving the bedroom windows wide open while the baby slept and his wife countered by bundling the infant to keep her warm. The baby died of crib suffocation, a sad event that placed a severe strain of recrimination and remorse on the marriage.

The greatest building blunder in Cragmor's long history of expansion occurred in the fall of 1929. The administration decided to construct a new nurses' home. Before that time the twenty-two nurses had been living in the cramped quarters of the Home or in small cubicles of the Main Building, lacking privacy and comfort. It now seemed advisable, reported Forster, to erect a large dormitory exclusively for the nurses. But the site was ill-chosen. Incomplete records divulge no information that a professional engineeer was called in to examine the bedrock, but a competent team of geologists might have persuaded Forster to avoid the costly and embarrassing disaster that ensued.

The building in question was a large, heavy, impressive structure four stories high, consisting of fifteen bedrooms with sleeping porches, several reception rooms, hardwood floors in each apartment, and a handsome mantelpiece and fireplace at one end of a spacious library. An attractive color scheme was varied for each room, only the best springs and mattresses were ordered, and every suite was wired for radio aerials. It promised to be the most elegant structure at Cragmor, built flush to the bluffs directly behind the Main Building, facing the south to afford a splendid view of the valley. Formal opening of this $60,000 home was held on July 27, 1930.[20] Shortly after its dedication the nurses joyously moved in, totally oblivious to the fact that the building had already begun to inch its way down the bluff, its foundation crumbling and cracking ever so slowly under the weight of a concrete mass supported by soft bentonite clay.

Before long, giant cracks appeared. The huge structure began to shudder. Doors jammed, water pipes burst, and the once-level floors tipped southward. Quickly the nurses, the furnishings, and all salvageable materials were removed. Then the inglorious new edifice was sealed up, condemned for further use. The debacle was quietly ignored. Not even *Ninety-Eight-Six* discussed the structural fiasco, the forced evacuation of its dwellers, or the plans to have it razed. The building was simply closed up and left abandoned for many years. The Cragmor nurses' home signaled the end of the empire-building era. In a sense its sudden demise epitomized as well the beginning of an epoch of seedy retreat from glory. Stone ruins lie on the hillside behind the Main Building today, a grim and easily overlooked reminder that stately palaces, like palatial dreams, will stand only as long as their base is sound.

It was quickly becoming apparent that Cragmor's base was not very sound any longer. The fall of 1929 brought even more problems. In the late afternoon of one October day a woman named Winifred J. Ackley fell down a sharp flight of stairs in the Main Building. She had misjudged the similarity of two doors. One opened onto a hallway leading to the ladies' room, where she expected to go; the other opened onto a platform from which a cement stairwell plunged into the abyss of Cragmor's furnace room, and it was there that she landed. A schoolteacher from Caldwell, Ohio, Mrs. Ackley had arrived at Cragmor the day before with deep asthmatic congestion, acute pulmonary tuberculosis, and severe headaches. She had just emerged from undergoing a series of X-ray examinations to help determine the extent of phthisical damage. Her tumble into Cragmor's cellar did little to lift her spirits or improve her health. In addition to a fractured spine and a broken ankle incurred by the fall, she later claimed that the three doctors who found her whimpering in a heap on the cellar floor exacerbated her injuries when they carried her back up the basement stairway. Accordingly, nineteen months later, when Mrs. Ackley was able to hobble into a Denver courthouse with her attorney, she filed a damage suit for $52,000 against the sanatorium for the cellar mishap and another $102,500 against Drs. Forster, McCrossin, and Good "for asserted mistreatment of her injuries."[21]

The lawsuit represented the familiar last straw on the proverbial camel's back for Cragmor's growing insolvency. It was discovered that the institution carried several unpaid insurance premiums, was remiss in paying back taxes, and had incurred a bonded indebtedness that could not be satisfied even by the seizure of a $50,000 insurance policy on the life of Dr. Gerald B. Webb and two $25,000 policies on the life of Dr. Alexius

Forster. Like the nation in the early throes of the Depression, Cragmor too began to reel in a fateful economic tailspin. Further investigations revealed that the management had defaulted in extending the property abstract and had failed to file answers to legal complaints. The upshot of the inquiry was the public announcement on November 24, 1935, of a foreclosure proceeding against the Cragmor Sanatorium. The institution was bankrupt.[22]

Subsequent early court action threatened to wrest Cragmor from local control and place it in the hands of eastern interests through a sheriff's sale. At one juncture it was rumored that a prominent New Yorker, whose name was not disclosed, had offered to buy the sanatorium; later it was reported that the prospective purchaser was in reality the Federal Emergency Relief Administration.[23]

As for Mrs. Ackley, she was awarded only one hundred dollars plus "other good and valuable considerations." On July 26, 1935, she died of galloping tuberculosis and complications arising from her accident at Cragmor. Though the judgment was unfavorable to her cause, the proceeding brought against the sanatorium, born of her fall, was the catalyst that presaged ill tidings for an institution already severely crippled by mismanagement and a general economic upheaval.

Cragmor's only outside support of ongoing and predictable funding came from an automatic trust known as the Mason C. Davidge Endowment, established in 1931 by David Randall MacIver of New York City in memory of his late brother-in-law, Mason Davidge, who had been a resident of Colorado Springs and a patient at Cragmor. The fund was intended to provide money for invalids of any background who required financial aid. Yet this single endowment, while generous, was a paltry sum compared to the enormous indebtedness of $600,000 incurred by Forster's bankrupt health resort and it too would be lost if the foreclosure hearing spelled the end to Cragmor's tenuous existence.

All seemed lost. Forster stood on the brink of losing his job, the patients and the staff were concerned about the future of their health care and employment, and the prospects of continuing to operate Cragmor as a private tubercular center seemed bleak indeed. But then, at the last moment, with a gesture reminiscent of a deus ex machina salvation scene on the classical stage, or the mounted stranger who rides his white steed into town to resolve insoluble difficulties, a benefactor stepped forward. His name was Robert Rhea, a one-time patient at Cragmor whose illness had been diagnosed as one of the worst ever treated at the asylum. He was now a healthy and prosperous Colorado Springs businessman, and was determined to extricate Cragmor from its financial plight in repayment for the excellent medical treatment that he had received under Dr. Forster's care.[24] Rhea quickly summoned all of the defendants, organized a bondholder's protective committee, satisfied creditors with payments from his own savings, and helped to absolve Forster and Cragmor's medical staff of personal indebtedness. The institution was then reorganized as a nonprofit, nonsectarian body called the Cragmor Foundation, "created for benevolent, charitable and humanitarian purposes and for the treatment of tuberculosis and other ailments."[25]

With its long trial of financial privation over, Cragmor enjoyed a short season of restored dignity. Some former patients rejoined the ranks of a dwindling population, prompting the local press to speak promisingly of "a revival of interest in bringing to this region persons of wealth and influence."[26] But in general the majority of Cragmor's invalids, reduced now in numbers from 185 to less than 60, continued to be those of limited means and advanced ailments. One example was the returnee Andrés Herrera, who in 1912 had spent nine months chasing the cure as one of Cuba's wealthiest emigrés. Since returning to Havana he had lost his oil and ranch business, contracted malaria, suffered a relapse of pulmonary tuberculosis, and been shot in the right nostril while being mugged one night. He was readmitted to Cragmor in 1932, utterly exhausted. A difficult patient, Herrera was impoverished but proud. Though he refused to buy his own thermometer, he nonetheless paid for the best private room service with money donated by friends.[27]

The institution's most crucial loss was the departure of Gerald Webb. Webb's labors as research director of the Colorado Foundation for Research in Tuberculosis, which he had organized in May of 1924, now demanded all of his time and professional energies.[28] One of his last benevolent gestures before leaving

Cragmor was to present the institution with the flagpole that still stands in front of the Main Building, plus three large poplars, "the Three Sentinels," on the edge of the front lawn. "When Dr. Webb departed," said one former patient, "it was like the end of a calm and beautiful day. His presence seemed always to give the place a touch of elegance and hope."[29] Another observer reported that "the age of dissatisfaction began when Gerald Webb left Cragmor. Thereafter it became a murky little hovel of insidious gossip, pettiness, sexual permissiveness, and neurotic disorders."[30]

In the course of its final year of publication, the institutional magazine, *Ninety-Eight-Six*, revealed some of the dismay that had begun to settle over the sanatorium. One individual, choosing to remain "forever anonymous," labeled the malady "Sanatoriosis," a condition that he described as "a warped outlook on life, a misguided philosophy which will not be to the advantage of patients." He suggested that the best weapon for combating "this serious and devastating disease, as deadly as its propagator, Tuberculosis," was "a good, well-developed sense of humor." Others too were disgruntled by Cragmor's melancholia. "Dr. Forster's warm greetings were becoming less effusive," said one employee. "He was a troubled man, and his personal gloom cast a mantle of sadness on the entire establishment."[31]

Much of Cragmor's cheerless climate could also be attributed to the fatalistic attitude that some patients had adopted concerning their minimal progress. The death rate reached its apex between 1936 and 1940, as did the rate of decline of the sanatorium's dwellers. Among the survivors were many human ruins, people too seriously ill to care about institutional morale. Conditions at Cragmor were really no different from those at other state hospitals. In January of 1931 a team of legislators, having begun a three-year investigation of Colorado's tubercular care problems only two years before, reported that their findings thus far indicated "an inadequate system of health administration throughout the state." One in every eight cases of tuberculosis ended in the patient's death. The report revealed that consumption was a definite threat to residents. Of 10,389 known cases of tuberculosis in Colorado in 1929, 5,690 or 54 percent were residents of the state.[32]

This ominous survey offered little cheer to anyone in the state stricken with TB and less comfort to Cragmorites, where the mortality rate, though somewhat better than one in eight, was still no lower than 10 percent. "The bodies were taken away at dawn, one every fortnight, sometimes three a month," observed a nurse who worked the night shift in 1934. "The mortician came in quietly and took away the deceased before anyone was awake. Yet somehow everyone knew he had been there. The following day people were silent and depressed."[33] One ex-patient of the era referred to Cragmor as "a depopulated island beyond the River Styx."[34]

A few improvements on the grounds gave the asylum a momentary facelift during the early thirties. A new laundry unit was built behind the garage, several trees were planted along the roadway, and an attractive lily pond appeared in front of the Main Building. But gradually the property showed signs of deterioration. The steam-heated greenhouse closed down in 1935, the gardens became overrun with weeds by the spring of 1936, and Dr. Houck's charming pathway had all but crumbled away through disuse by 1937. "Dad" White, the eccentric old caretaker, died in the midthirties; his replacements were deemed "slovenly, lecherous men who augmented scandal."[35] Despite "Dad" White's gruff exterior and strange fetish for gathering buttons out of garbage cans—an enterprise to which he devoted most of his spare time—he had kept the sanatorium grounds immaculate. His death was a harbinger of the forties: rot, refuse, and rats.

Internal dissatisfaction increased. With the disbanding of *Ninety-Eight-Six*, the eight-year-long tradition of showing weekly motion pictures in the dining room, supported by the magazine's proceeds, was also discontinued. That event signaled the end of organized social programming for the guests.

During the winter months of 1931–32 complaints circulated in the Home that radios could not be properly heard owing to transmission interference. It was soon discovered that a proliferation of electric blankets was the cause. Many patients were "bundling" in new, large-sized bedwarmers. Forster immediately forbade the use of all electrical heating apparatuses, not to improve radio reception, but because the illicit pads and blankets ran counter to Cragmor's time-honored fresh-air philosophy of total exposure to the elements. After the electric blanket ban, however, radios blared so loudly that their incessant playing had to be curbed. Cragmor's "radio menace" was then so strongly denounced by Forster that by mid-1933 he made it a point to ask each new patient to subscribe bountifully to magazines "and other quiet distractions," leaving "all objects of noise" at home.[36]

Despite the ever-tightening strain on the local economy, one patient made his personal fortune at Cragmor. Chase Stone, who had been confined at Cragmor since 1924, began a lucrative enterprise in the fall of 1931, a "bed-side hobby" as he called it, which provided the catalyst for his life's work. As the sanatorium's residential consultant for Boettcher-Neuton Brokerage, Stone went from room to room and from rooftop to dining hall to garden, acquainting patients, employees, and the staff with his service. Stone offered stock-beleaguered invalids a genuine panacea for their sorrow over the crash of 1929: a reassuring smile and sound financial advice. During his last years at Cragmor, Chase Stone became one of the retreat's most wealthy patients, simply by having assisted fellow lungers with their stock and bond investments. "Chase was a charming, personable chap," stated Rabbi Kopald. "He always had an optimistic word about the market and the nation's financial scene; but more importantly, he had the know-how to deal with people. If Chase Stone made a fortune at Cragmor, it was an honest one, and it was only because people loved him and trusted him with their money."[37]

The Cragmor of the thirties was not without an occasional luminary to excite local hero-worshipers. The most prominent figure was Vincent Youmans (1898–1946), one of America's most prolific composers of musical comedy scores during the previous decade. Shortly after completing his score for the Ginger Rogers/Fred Astaire film, *Flying Down to Rio*, Youmans collapsed of exhaustion. The intensity with which he had been working since his London debut of *No, No, Nanette* eight years before, coupled with the trauma of a divorce, affected his health. At the insistence of his physicians, Youmans retired to Colorado Springs for a rest cure. He had made half a million dollars by the age of twenty-seven, writing such songs as "Tea For Two" and "I Want to be Happy," but he looked aged, drawn, and impoverished upon his arrival at Cragmor. You-mans spent many months in veritable seclusion, emerging from his suite from time to time late at night, long after the rest of the sanatorium had retired, to play quietly on the grand piano in the dining hall. Cragmor marked for Youmans the beginning of a long ten-year hiatus during which he was unable to write or publish any new songs.[38]

Residing in a private suite just down the hall from Youmans was a strange personality, generally shrouded in shawls, a middle-aged dancer from Russia known as Madame Snjinski. Once the dancing partner of Pavlova, this stocky and often crabby woman considered herself the empress of the sanatori-um. She insisted on tray service, drank only goat's milk, spoke lovingly of Leo Tolstoy, and somehow managed to whistle mel-odies by Tchaikowsky through her nose. She was a fidgety and temperamental guest "with a frightful exterior," reported one nurse. "She succeeded in alienating most of her fellow in-mates."[39]

Another difficult patient was Felix Doubleday of the famed publishing clan. Aloof and intolerant of other patients' concerns, he spent many hours by himself polishing his valuable brass and copper statuettes. He once phoned the kitchen to order a fig and prune laxative known as "food of the gods." A woebegone kitchen maid understood Doubleday to say "food for my dogs." When she entered his suite carrying a dish with grissle and bones, all hell broke loose. Doubleday was not amused and the poor maid suffered a brutal tongue-lashing.[40]

As of February 13, 1936, owing to Robert Rhea's benevolent intervention on Cragmor's behalf, the new sanatorium was fully incorporated and began operating as a servant of the public. It had surrendered its thirty-year title as a privately owned asy-lum; profits or taxes would no longer trouble its management—so it was believed. The board of directors first met in March of 1936 to acknowledge a gift of one thousand dollars from the new savior and benefactor, Robert Rhea, and to approve a sub-stantial loan from its intrepid helmsman, Dr. Alexius M. Forster.[41] In later meetings the foundation agreed to pay the res-ident physicians a modest monthly salary of one hundred dol-lars each, although within one year of that decision those same doctors were asked to release the foundation from that obligation and to accept a token reduction in wages, owing to the corporation's sudden plunge into financial instability.[42] Soon the body's penury increased to such an extent that by December of 1938 the foundation decided to rent out a large portion of Cragmor's vacant buildings to pay off its enormous debts.[43]

As the thirties dragged to a close amidst the horrors of a new war in Europe, the Cragmor Sanatorium was a mere tragi-grotesque shadow of its former glory. Its patients consisted of "a motley assortment," claims Mildred Russell, "from crude louts to fallen aristocrats. Generally they were too sick for much non-sense."[44] Whatever "nonsense" took place was restricted in the main to the ranks of management: carefree hanky-panky be-tween doctors and nurses, consultants in bed with patients, or nurses involved with employees. One individual had acquired an irrepressible reputation as the institution's gigolo; one of the greenhouse men, spending too little time with his tulip bulbs, was dismissed for homosexuality; another gardener was threat-ened by fellow employees into marrying the orphan lass he had abused; and so it went. . . . Low wages, improvised entertain-ment, furtive drinking, and a quiet death—these were the hall-marks of Cragmor's declining years.

In the forties, the splendor that was once the mighty Cragmor sank ever deeper into the mire. Much was due to Alexius For-ster's unfortunate decline. As Forster slumped heavily into a disabling mental disorder, his managerial energies spent by the mounting vexations of personal and professional concerns, the institution that he had engineered since 1910 became, in the words of a former nurse "a dirty, dark, and dreary place."[45] It was so run-down by 1941, in fact, that public health inspectors had to be summoned from Colorado Springs to enforce minimal standards of hygiene. Pack rats invaded the kitchen by night, insects and mice by day; sewage lines were left unrepaired; roaches infested the bedding; pigeons roosted in the broken sleeping porch awnings; the buildings, pathways, and gardens fell into a state of decay and abandon. One former employee re-lates that the front lawn was so badly neglected that it turned to weeds. "We were told not to sit on the grass, or what was left of it, because rattlesnakes were so plentiful." In brief, Cragmor was a dismal, ugly dump.

"The patients left Cragmor in a worse condition than when

they came," was one former nurse's observation. "It was no longer a fashionable care center; it wasn't even a decent hospital. It was a rubbish heap of the most appalling deterioration." During the summer of 1942 there was one stretch of three consecutive weeks when custodial services were completely suspended. It was then that a night-duty nurse threw up from the stench of a fourth-floor closet she had opened. There before her were three-foot-high piles of filthy sputum cups, stained with dry mucous. One elderly female patient, left unattended in a darkened reception hall, suffered a massive hemorrhage as she stumbled from room to room screaming for her nurse. "She banged on my door," stated her neighbor down the hall. "I opened it and stood looking at her in horror. Her lips were gummed together, and out of her throat, instead of words, came a strange rattling noise. She grabbed her side and fell head first into my room, dead." Another old woman reportedly killed herself "rather than spend another day suffering in that squalor." The early forties, relates one ex-Cragmorite, were "a time of confusion at Cragmor. Most of the invalids were a pathetic sight to behold—gaunt, dirty, in extreme misery. . . . Many of them, especially the Mexican and Indian patients, were badly neglected or mistreated." According to four other individuals, several members of Cragmor's medical staff were too involved with young nurses or with their live-in mistresses to care much for the welfare of the patients. One Cragmorite affirms that the only constant diversion in the Main Building was "extra-marital bed-hopping on every floor." Another confirms this report, adding that at the time of Forster's mental breakdown (1947), Cragmor was a "scene of disorder and rampant sex."

The most telling illustration of debauchery was the case of a young female patient nicknamed Dottie, "pale like the angel of phthisis," who conducted secret nocturnal orgies with her doctor. Her antics prompted a kind of sensual hysteria among three jealous inmates lodging nearby. One night they ensconced themselves in her room, one under the bed and two in the wardrobe. Their vicarious pleasure was thwarted, however, when a coughing fit seized one of the curious spies. As a result of the misadventure, Dottie suffered convulsions, providing her doctor friend with more work than he had bargained for.

On the pretext of taking a baby because the mother was tuberculous, many abortions were performed at the Cragmor Sanatorium between 1941 and 1947. An ex-nurse who assisted at some of the operations refers to the sanatorium as "the abortion center of Colorado Springs." Another dates her own inauguration as a nurse's aide at Cragmor from the time she attended the extraction of a human fetus. She was told that her medical career would be finished if she ever reported the incident. "Local doctors would drive out to Cragmor with young, unwed, pregnant girls," she relates. "The girls were admitted as 'incipient tuberculars.' A few days later they were released to go home, cured." Another ex-nurse attests that "were the true facts known about Cragmor's abortion program, it would tarnish the reputation of some of the community's finest families."[46]

By September of 1947 this clandestine operation came to an abrupt end. Perhaps someone blew the whistle or threatened legal action. In an emergency session of the board of directors of the Cragmor Foundation, all "therapeutic correctments," as the abortion enterprise was euphemistically termed, were sharply condemned: "Such treatment is to be positively and definitely stopped," state the minutes.[47] Fortunately for the Cragmor asylum's continuing operation, the issue was never made public. The subsequent cover-up extended to the destruction of classified medical records and to the intimidation of nursing collaborators. The fear of scandal could not have benefited Forster's precarious nervous state. Immediately following the motion to halt abortions at Cragmor, he requested and was granted a leave of absence "for an indefinite period."[48]

Until its reorganization in 1936, Cragmor had always managed to proffer medical care exclusively for America's commonweal of the stricken lung, those young men and women whose education or professional ambitions were halted by the dreadful tubercle bacilli. Occasionally, of course, asthma or even chronic hay fever may have been misdiagnosed as incipient tuberculosis, so quite unintentionally a nontuberculous individual could enter the sanatorium in that era. However, consumption was the only disease actually treated. Now, however, under the new corporate charter it was possible for the sanatorium's staff to treat other ailments besides tuberculosis, though the name or nature of the other diseases remained undefined on the patients' records. In the spring of 1943, however, one of the unclassified other ailments clearly included the treatment of syphilis, a disease as common as the Great White Plague among the large entourage of male patients who entered Cragmor representing the Grand Lodge of the Brotherhood of Railroad Trainmen from Cleveland, Ohio. It was the sanatorium's stated policy with respect to the railroad invalids to treat venereal disease "with conservatism and the avoidance of all radical measures."[49] Furthermore, it was agreed by Cragmor's board of directors that the term syphilis would be vigorously avoided and excluded from all official medical documents.

The syphilitic railroad employees, some of whom were unquestionably tuberculous, were restricted at first to closed quarters within the Main Building. They were charged eighty-five dollars per month per patient for room, board, and medical treatment, and were ordered to avoid any contact with Cragmor's female population. As their venereal symptoms abated, the men were permitted to eat in the dining room and to socialize with the other patients, but only in groups. Cragmor's contract with the Cleveland outfit gave the asylum a substantial financial boost. Within two years the institution's population had nearly doubled and its assets had more than tripled.

The war effort abroad and the natural hazards of living at Cragmor prompted the foundation to order the razing of two abandoned buildings late in 1942. Because of the scarcity of critical materials needed for ammunition and war machinery—principally iron and copper tubing—both the nurses' home, deserted from the time of its ignominious closure ten years before, and the Cragmor power plant, no longer operable, were torn down.[50] The nurses' home was deemed a special menace as long as it stood against the bluff, cracking, sliding, and splintering with each passing year. All of the cottages within a one-half block radius of the condemned monstrosity had to be abandoned "because of the danger that it might fall and injure someone."[51] The old cabins themselves were so dilapidated that renters who chose to live there did so at their own risk. They were required, in fact, to sign a release of liability for any damage or death "which might occur in their occupancy."[52]

Like the unstable structures they lived in, Cragmor's patients were a generally sorry lot. The lungers of the 1940s were a far cry from their elegant predecessors of the affluent past. Gone were the Billings, the Pulitzers, the Doubledays, the Cowles, the immortal Youmans, the legendary Chase Stone. Gone were the cosmopolitan playboys chasing flamboyant maidens, the prosperous lungers gliding in private planes, the pajama-clad hedonists drinking cocktails on the front lawn, the late-night bridge players and early-dawn croquet enthusiasts, the high-rolling gamblers and adventuresome bootleggers, the well-tanned backsides lingering with the last rays of a Colorado sunset on the luxuriant roof garden. By 1942, old Cragmor had degenerated into a second-rate clinic for sometime-tuberculars. It was only half-filled with impoverished local invalids, a handful of distraught Navajo Indians, ten frightened Mexican farmers, some twenty or more syphilitic railroad men, and a dozen miscellaneous lungers—none eager to stay long, all hoping to survive for just one more day.

And nothing much happened. Like T. S. Eliot's J. Alfred Prufrock, who measured out his life with coffee spoons, Cragmor's quiet chasers counted their days by the monotonous red and black markings on the "temp and sputum" charts. Their lives consisted of fevers, a coughing siege, rest hours, and tolerable meals. A few died, some languished with dreadful suffering, but most of them went home again, overjoyed to leave Cragmor and all that it represented.

The late forties into the early fifties were the saddest of all sad years at Cragmor. Then the unprosperous asylum became the refuge for a brigade of World War II veterans. It was the time when Forster was obliged to resign his post as medical director and seek psychiatric help at Brady's Hospital. It was also the time when Brooks D. Good, the affable but ailing doctor who temporarily replaced Forster, suddenly died. They were bleak years, years of frustration, pain, and death.

The first major difficulty arose during the final year of Forster's command. Labor disputes erupted between disgruntled employees and management. Charges of an overbearing work routine were leveled at Forster. The kitchen help requested more vacation time, tray boys demanded overtime compensation, and room maids asked for improved working hours. As a result of these complaints and protests, the Cragmor Foundation formally established a two-week vacation with pay for all employees and granted a six-day-week contract to every individual on the payroll. It also approved the hiring of an assistant for Forster, shortly before his resignation. Forster's many duties seemed to have become a taxing burden to his tentative sense of well-being.[53]

A second problem ensued with the arrival in February of 1947 of fifty boisterous veterans from Denver's overcrowded Fitzsimons Hospital. Cragmor's New Building was turned over to the Veterans Administration, a fortuitous event for stimulating the fiscal lifeline of the aging health resort but signaling trouble for a number of threatened inmates among Cragmor's resident male population. These men resented the fact that the limited nursing staff would henceforth be obliged to attend to the frivolous needs of a regiment of lusty vets.[54] For their part, the veterans were delighted to be at Cragmor. Here they could receive more personal care in an environment of less confusion and less authoritarian rule than that of the mammoth, dehumanized Fitzsimons. And they were especially fond of Cragmor's young medical attendants and female employees. They moved freely about the sanatorium, making friends, courting, gambling, and singing. In short, they fully enjoyed their civilian-centered convalescence.

On one occasion a fist fight erupted in the dining hall when a group of ex-soldiers made amorous advances on several young ladies. Their consumptive male friends took offense. The incident induced several of the badly mauled patients to write angry letters to Fitzsimons Hospital requesting that the villainous vets be transferred back to Denver "for conduct unbecoming the nation's military." A carload of commanding officers and medical staff visited Cragmor and agreed to expel the vets; however, Senators Johnson and Millikan, Representative Chenoweth, and the Veterans Administration Post No. 5 of the American Legion rallied to the veterans' cause. They successfully persuaded the Fitzsimons review board to allow Cragmor's ex-service lads to remain in Colorado Springs.[55]

The third and most telling dilemma was Forster's alarming decline and breakdown. Once a peppery, witty, carefree individual, Forster had entered the thirties as a temperamental and difficult man to deal with. Some remember him as "overbearing and cantankerous," others as "a man beset with worry," and "a churlish sort constantly on edge." As he approached his fifty-

fifth year of age, Forster's strength had been drained by the con-
tinous stress of financial woes. His once buoyant spirit now
showed signs of wilting. He became increasingly listless and
unresponsive, more the grumpy taskmaster of a penal colony
than the jocose patriarch of that rules-free resort that he had
fashioned into a world-renowned sanatorium.

Forster's deterioration symbolized the end of a golden era at
the Colorado health resort. As Cragmor's dizzy prosperity vanished, leaving in its wake a swelling financial crisis, so too did
its once dapper and energetic leader crumble into a state of
weariness and confusion. His clothes looked old, shabby, and
dirty. He was frequently seen shuffling along dark corridors late
at night, turning off lights, unscrewing bulbs, closing doors,
talking half-aloud to himself, and tripping over his own untied
shoelaces. He was gruff and short-tempered with the employees, suffered occasional memory lapses, and was said to be
overly fond of buttermilk laced with bourbon.[56]

For many years Forster had been living in the Main Building.
The home he had once occupied on Cragmor Road had been
sold in 1944 and he moved his French wife Liane and two
daughters into a Village cottage. The long years of separation
from his wife, first occasioned when their baby died of asfixia-
tion, had taken a heavy toll on Forster's health and stamina.
Then in the fall of 1947 a series of unfortunate incidents occurred between Forster and Cragmor's personnel, obliging the
other members of the board of directors to demand that Forster
"surrender his room and office at Cragmor Sanatorium and that
he stay off the premises of Cragmor Sanatorium until further order of the Board."[57]

Forster willingly entered the Emory John Brady Hospital for
psychiatric treatment on October 2, 1947. He remained there
through October 28. Later that year he applied to the Cragmor
Foundation for reinstatement, but the board refused to honor
his request, stating that both the medical report and a survey
taken of Cragmor's patients deemed it inadvisable.[58] In the
spring of 1948 he again petitioned for reinstatement, having secured the written support of four doctors to attest that he was
no longer a danger to himself or to others. Forster was thereby
readmitted as a voting member of the board of directors but he
was denied all managerial responsibilities at the sanatorium and

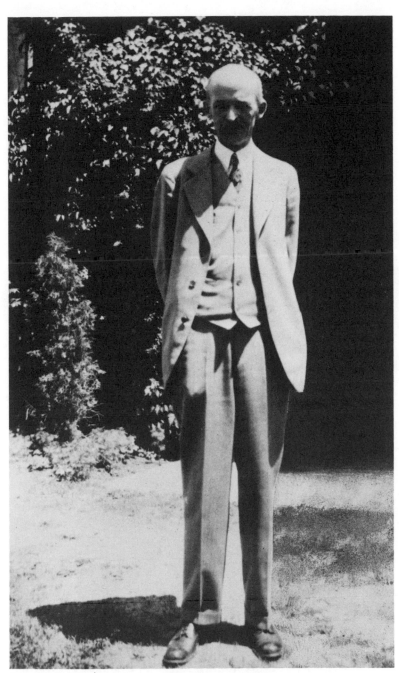

Forster in his final year as managing director

was reduced to serving as a part-time medical consultant under the direction of Dr. Brooks Good. "Dr. Forster shall exercise no authority in the finances or business management of the sanatorium" read the foundation's grim decree.[59] He was permitted to examine patients or X-rays, but was required to submit a written report of any case he handled to Dr. Good.

It was a sad and humiliating mandate to impose on the very man who had presided over the growth and splendor, as well as the decline, of the Cragmor Sanatorium for thirty-seven years. Forster accepted the verdict—he really had no choice if he wished to remain on the sanatorium's payroll. The foundation agreed to pay him a salary of $250 per month, the same amount that he had been receiving as the medical director. The old helmsman, weary of the struggle, moved to town and for a brief time enjoyed the companionship of his trusted friend, Nell Coxwell, who looked after him.[60] But in 1950 Nell left for California, leaving the seventy-year-old physician bereft, broken-hearted, and alone.

A new psychiatric examination in 1953 dispelled suspicions of senility and put to rest the rumors of a permanent mental disorder. "It is my opinion," wrote Dr. E. James Brady, apropos of Forster's wish to be fully reinstated at Cragmor, "that he does not, at this time, suffer from a disabling mental disease. If he returns to work, it is my recommendation that he not be given administrative responsibility, and that his clinical responsibilities be limited in such a way as to avoid undue emotional strain which might again precipitate a recurrence of his former mental illness."[61]

Forster's last year at Cragmor was an unpleasant experience. While a few old friends treated him with respect and some with veneration, others passed him by as a quaint relic of the past. To the end, however, Forster remained congenial and cooperative, displaying no animosity toward those whose deportment he had blamed for provoking earlier fits of wrath and the aggravation of his hypomanic state. He shuffled about the sanatorium, reminiscing with older patients over his empire days at Cragmor.

On Tuesday, March 23, 1954, Alexius M. Forster died at the age of seventy-three. Six months later the Cragmor Foundation hung a plaque in his memory in the lobby of the sanatorium.

The board of directors drafted a brief resolution to honor his service at Cragmor:

> Through the long years of difficulties and adversities the courage, perseverance, and devotion of Doctor Forster has been an unfaltering beacon which has guided the Foundation to its present position.
>
> His devotion and services to the Foundation have been of inestimable value and the loss occasioned by his death will long be felt. Adversity after adversity have been encountered and overcome, and as the Foundation now approaches a greater fulfillment of its purposes, Doctor Forster would have derived much satisfaction from the part which his devotion and services played in aiding the Foundation to the complete realization of these purposes.[62]

Several years later the Forster plaque disappeared, apparently the victim of theft. By then the sanatorium had dwindled in size. Ten years after his death, the Cragmor Foundation was dissolved and the once-proud health resort closed its doors, the last institution of its kind in the state of Colorado. Thereafter the name Cragmor would be nothing more than a misspelled entry on city maps (Cragmore), designating a small residential community on the north end of town.

Yet before it closed its doors, there would be one more chapter to the Cragmor story, a welcome lift from the depths to which the sanatorium had fallen.

SIX

The Navajo Indian Decade

*You are not on vacation. You
are here to get well. Try to get
along with everyone and stay
away from men.*
                    Annie Wauneka

The first Indian patients to enter Cragmor under the United
States government contract of 1952 were flown from Window
Rock, Arizona, in an old Tripacer airplane. They were part of a
massive health program launched under the auspices of the
Bureau of Indian Affairs and later controlled by a division of the
newly created Department of Health, Education, and Welfare.
Cragmor was one of the initial fifteen contract institutions for
the care of tuberculous Indians. When the program ended, it
was one of the last to close.

Long before the United States government subsidized Cragmor's final decade of operation, there had been several small
bands of Indian patients admitted to the sanatorium. The first
group came during the early months of the Depression—all migratory charity cases. Later, clusters of Navajos drifted in to
seek health care under the institution's only benevolent endowment, the Mason Davidge Fund. According to the insect-
nibbled, water-smudged records of that era, the first Navajo
lungers were extremely ill. Several of them died at Cragmor,
most were listed in critical condition, and very few were
released before two years of hospitalization. How these hapless
Indians had come to land at Cragmor remains one of the least
studied yet most fascinating chapters of modern regional lore.
The general facts involve one of Colorado's most enterprising
con artists, the legendary flim-flam medicine man and soldier of
fortune Doctor Yosemite Nabona.[1]

Late in the year 1928, Nabona and his wife emigrated from Miami Beach to Colorado Springs. A Florida hurricane had decimated Nabona's southern base of operation, so he heeded the advice of a friend who suggested that "Colorado was the land of suckers" and set up his log cabin community on a two-acre tract located on the southern edge of the Black Forest, just off Templeton Gap Road. This first structure was a mysterious factory where secret herbs were brewed and curative Indian rites performed.

Nabona was known far and wide as the Indian Doctor, a suitable epithet for a man who himself was a full-blooded Navajo and who catered to the needs of itinerant Indian consumptives. At a time when tuberculosis struck one out of every three Navajo families and Navajo babies were dying in appalling numbers from diarrhea caused by spoiled canned milk, Nabona's magic formulas and winsome personality attracted hundreds of desperate Indian mothers to his Black Forest sanatorium.

His own parents had died of tuberculosis on a government reservation at Red House, Arizona, and Nabona was left an orphan at the age of nine. For a few years young Yosemite lived with foster parents, a German couple who ran a modest farm in the Texas Panhandle. They later adopted him and then sold their farm and moved back to their native Germany. Yosemite enrolled at the University of Berlin and graduated with a degree in medicine. He also acquired a portly frame and a burning desire to see the world. He left Germany, never to return.

Nabona drifted from mercenary military service into self-trained fakir work. First he fought for the United States at the battle of Manila, then with the Boers in South Africa, and later as a member of the French Foreign Legion in North Africa. He then served in the Mexican navy, studied aboriginal medicine along the Amazon River, and practiced Hindu ascetic rites in India. It was in Calcutta that Doctor Nabona learned the mysterious arts, chants, and quackery that he later put to use in Colorado.

Nabona was a gigantic man—some say he weighed over three hundred pounds. He drank large quantities of liquor, lavished charm across the Seven Seas, married a lovely white woman whom he had once cured with his own secret blend of moss and barley, and ultimately built a lucrative empire on buncombe and balderdash north of Colorado Springs.

He called his settlement the Navajo Indian Village. It was incorporated under the rapidly expanding umbrella of the widely advertised Navajo Indian Remedies Company of which Yosemite Nabona was sole proprietor. He claimed to have colonies and agencies throughout the United States and in many foreign countries. His business grew so rapidly in the summer of 1928 that the proverbial path was beaten to his door. Observers counted as many as seventy-five automobiles parked at his Black Forest settlement at one time. He boasted of having treated as many as seven hundred patients in one day and spent more than $60,000 in one year to develop his log cabin health spa.[2]

If high winds had blown him out of Florida, his own hot air, coupled with the nation's numbing economic collapse in 1929, forced Nabona to close the Rocky Mountain branch of his health cure enterprise. In the final months of its operation several Navajo families, most of them tuberculous, earned their keep by compounding Nabona's mystical remedies, selling basketwork to visitors, and attracting hundreds of tourists and fellow consumptives to the site, all of whom willingly paid the required fee for a chance to see Dr. Nabona at work in his famous laboratory and medicine factory. Though local doctors assailed his business, warning patients against "illusory conjurations," Nabona made a fortune on the gullibility of the trusting lungers who stayed to chase the cure at his popular magic show. When the exposition folded, some of the Indian Doctor's diseased victims, having no place else to go, transferred their quest for a miracle cure to the vine–laden walls of Cragmor Sanatorium. Small clusters of disappointed invalids, some of them Anglo, most of them Mexican and Indian migrants, filtered piecemeal into Glockner, Sunnyrest, and Cragmor, seeking charitable health care.

Forster and his staff took in as many of Nabona's refugees as Cragmor could accommodate, but with perceptible misgivings. The downtrodden patients, after all, offered nothing to improve the name, stature, or fiscal fabric of their new-found beneficent home. Some of Cragmor's other patients remember them as pathetic, critically diseased, socially crippled, and grievously alienated human beings. "If they didn't die of tuberculosis," remarked an ex–lunger, "they surely must have perished from neglect and loneliness."[3] Another observed: "Cragmor was like a prison in those days, and the poor Navajo and Mexican vagrants made up its ward of solitary confinement."[4]

It was a strikingly different group of Navajos that entered Cragmor two decades later. The Nabona stragglers had all passed away or had sought refuge elsewhere by 1952, leaving the sanatorium's suites all the more desolate, emptied of even its surplus charity cases. Feelings of obsolescence then gripped the hospital. The staff spoke in sad, hushed tones of ominous days ahead; George Dwire, the director, pondered the feasibility of securing a new contract with the Brotherhood of Railroad Trainmen; the foundation's directors lamented that their cash on hand had plummeted to a mere $25,000, the only money available to support the continuing operation of a cure center crying out for many needed repairs.[5]

Then in November of 1952 the United States government entered into a contract with Cragmor and fourteen other western hospitals and sanatoriums, guaranteeing the institution a permanent base of financial support in exchange for its willingness to administer to the medical needs of hundreds of tuberculous Navajos. Approximately seventy patients, flown in from Arizona and New Mexico, were the first Indians to be admitted to Cragmor in the 1950s. "They literally saved the place from slow strangulation," reported C. J. Munro, president of the Cragmor Foundation.[6] Until the government contract went into effect, sponsored by the Indian Service Division of the Department of the Interior, the nearly deserted cure house that Solly had built was well on its way to a final state of bankruptcy. Now, all at once the sanatorium's population jumped from twenty to ninety patients. And with the government providing a per diem payment of $11.75 per Navajo, Cragmor's income automatically increased by nearly $25,000 during the first year of the Indian contract. Under the perceptive management of George Dwire, who was constantly struggling with all income, investment, salary, and spending problems, the Cragmor Foundation's assets swelled to $404,257 by the end of 1955, only three years after the Navajo program had begun.[7]

For nearly a decade Cragmor was again a thriving and even

respectable care center. The foundation had sufficient money to grant annuities to Frieda Lochthowe, the head nurse; to George Dwire, the managing director; and to several staff assistants. Employees' salaries were measurably increased; within one brief period of eighteen months, some of them doubled. Costly improvements could now be paid for in cash. In 1956 the foundation hired a chief engineer named Mel Reiner, who was charged with overseeing the maintenance and improvements of the refurbished physical plant. He was paid $400 per month for his services. Later that year the Ford Foundation granted Cragmor a gift of $47,000, earmarked for the purchase of new furniture and medical equipment.[8]

By early 1958 the foundation's capital funds were so abundant that Dwire could report the availability of a quarter of a million dollars which, when matched by an equal amount in federal funds promised under the Hill-Barton Act, would permit the construction of a modern nursing home attached to the Main Building. Plans for the luxurious edifice were immediately approved and the construction was begun without delay. Within two years the nursing home opened its doors for business. It was the last building to be erected in the history of the Cragmor Sanatorium. It bore the name Cragmor Manor.[9]

This, then, was the promising setting for Cragmor's swan song as a tubercular hospital. Federal monies abounded, the institution teemed with patients, and Navajo arts flourished. Once again the dining hall became an active recreation center. Patients crowded around television sets donated to the sanatorium by the El Pomar Center, attended the newly restored weekly movies, and played on the old grand piano, which had remained idle and out of tune for nearly two decades. A novelty shop opened on the fourth floor, school classes were conducted in the old Solly cabin, and one light and airy kitchen became the site for modern cooking instruction, food preparation, and basic dietary rules under the direction of Mildred Dawson.

Cragmor still maintained a small staff. The director, one house physician, half a dozen consultants, a personnel supervisor, ten nurses, and a handful of teachers promoted an atmosphere for creative learning and a pleasant convalescence in the once–somber suites. Only ten years earlier, the motto, "if you survive Cragmor, you'll survive anything," seemed to have

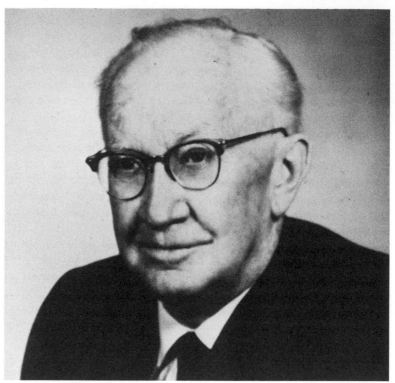

George T. Dwire

been the operable outlook. Now the new philosophy was Dwire's statement: "Rest the body, improve the mind, and let laughter abound."[10]

George T. Dwire, the managing director, was a dentist by profession, though for thirty years under the guidance of Gerald Webb and Alexius Forster he had gained valuable on-the-job training in tuberculosis care. He had first come to Cragmor in 1922 as one of Webb's patients. James R. Shaw, the man who spearheaded the Indian health program in the American Southwest, speaks of George Dwire as one of the most efficient and energetic directors he ever met: "He was an excellent physician and administrator who sincerely believed in what he was doing and who was intent on making a major contribution to the Indians. He deeply felt his obligations and provided a warm, welcome environment; he understood the cultural, social, economic, and nutritional problems of his patients; and he recognized the deep fundamental differences between the various tribes and clans. He made broad adjustments within his operation to make the various kinds of Indians feel comfortable, welcome, and happy."[11]

Under Dwire's direction Cragmor's medical services expanded to include educational and occupational therapy. The program was tailor-made to fit the needs of a diverse and culturally different group of people. Along with his chief of staff, Dr. Henry W. Maly, Dwire was credited for having hired a team of highly competent educators and nurses to provide the Indian women with the kind of psychological security that would prove most beneficial for their rapid recovery. Unlike the Navajos before them, who had languished throughout the Depression in a state of fear and loneliness, confined to the back rooms of the sanatorium, the Indians of the 1950s were contented and optimistic. No expense was spared to give them first-rate medical care, individualized instruction in elementary school subjects, and realistic leisure-time therapy. This attention enabled the Indian patients to work at their native crafts during the long days and months of convalescence.

Despite his many managerial accomplishments, George Dwire was not everybody's favorite personality. "He was a crusty, brash, and short-tempered man," said one Cragmorite. "If Doctor Forster was cold and aloof with the hired help, Doctor Dwire was downright ferocious!" claimed another.[12] "He was a very stubborn individual," reported a colleague, "stubborn, opinionated, and demanding, but, oh boy, could that man get the job done right!"[13] Some people, however, remember Dwire as a warm and personable gentleman, generous with his time, his money, and his talent. He wielded a powerful political clout in the state and much of Cragmor's advancement was directly attributable to his powers of persuasion in the governor's office. Having seen how the rich had always received favorable treatment at Cragmor during the early Forster years, Dwire lobbied energetically for the defeat of all anti-indigency bills in state-supported tubercular care. "He won those battles," explained one of the region's physicians, "because no one dared oppose him! He was a formidable adversary. I thanked Providence for the wisdom or good luck to be on his side in an argument."[14]

However much Dwire's public image may have fluctuated in the eyes of his colleagues or the asylum's hired help, the fact remains that he fostered a milieu of helpfulness, gentle understanding, and positive learning experiences among the Navajos. To this day many of those young patients, long since recovered, cherish his kindness to them. Shaw observes that the Cragmor of the fifties under George Dwire regained its former stature in the field of tuberculosis; it was again recognized as a first-rate resort operated "with vigor, imagination, and ingenuity."[15]

As Dwire stood for foresight and good judgment, a soft-spoken man named Otto Einstein, who served as the sanatorium's house physician for twelve years (1947-59), was the individual to whom hundreds of patients, employees, and nurses turned for comforting words of encouragement and medical advice. "Einstein was the most unassuming hero of Cragmor's medical faculty," reports one of his Cragmor Village patients.[16] His life before coming to Cragmor had been filled with heartache and rugged buffetings. For thirty-five years he had practiced pediatrics in Stuttgart, Germany, but then came Hitler and the Jewish purge. The aging doctor was given one of two choices: either the concentration camp or exile. He chose the latter, leaving his home and all his worldly possessions in the hands of the Nazi gestapo. For nine months he labored in Nicaragua as a missionary physician, then he secured an immigration visa to live in the United States. After spending five years at the Woodmen Sanatorium, retraining himself at the age of sixty-five to be a licensed surgeon, Einstein accepted a position at the troubled Cragmor Sanatorium at the very time the institution was passing through its abortion crisis. Einstein was, in fact, the man who eventually replaced Forster as Cragmor's resident physician when Forster requested an indefinite leave of absence in the wake of personal and professional problems.

Otto Einstein, a cousin and close friend of the famous Albert Einstein, devoted the last six years of his life to the many tuberculous Indians who had come to Cragmor under his care. "He was an intensely compassionate man," recalls one of the nurses who assisted him on his rounds. "He cared so deeply about people that he would sit for hours in vigil at the bedside of a terminally ill patient, just to convey that last word of comfort and assurance when no one else cared."[17] Another attendant reports that the Cragmor staff had planned a party for him on his eightieth birthday but Einstein was nowhere to be seen. "We were terribly worried that something had happened to him, so someone went from room to room searching for him, fearing he had died of a heart attack. He was discovered on the fourth floor, reading a Mother Goose book aloud to a group of entranced Navajo children."[18] Wherever sounds of laughter were heard, so the saying went, Otto Einstein could be found nearby.

He was a man of rigid, undeviating principles for himself, though greatly tolerant of others' mistakes. "Even the aspirin tablets taken home from the Sanatorium had to be paid for," wrote Rabbi Kaiman, "and the uncancelled stamps on letters overlooked by the postal authorities had to be torn up."[19] Once, when a nurse was scolding a youth for her refusal to swallow candy-coated medicine, Einstein sided with the patient. He escorted the pajama-clad youngster to his laboratory where together they carefully removed all of the dye and sugar-coating from her pills and added a solution to her liquid medicine to make it taste like cabbage. Thereafter, it was reported that the doctor's young patients stood in line at his laboratory waiting to have their medicine turned into cabbage juice. They would then swallow their sugarless medication with gusto.[20]

Einstein was once asked to care for a nursing attendant's cat. Having just completed his Colorado medical exam to practice surgery, the doctor was imbued with a desire to observe the animal more as a medical specimen than someone's beloved pet. When the aide returned from her short vacation and asked Einstein for the cat, the doctor was discombobulated. His avid curiosity had killed the cat. An interest in its mild sniffles had led to a complete biopsy. It took the cat's owner many years to realize that her cat-sitter was not a savage butcher, only a commited scientist whose interest in feline anatomy got the best of him.[21]

Except for the cat incident, the old gentleman was a beloved figure at Cragmor. Uprooted from a career of caring for children in southern Germany, renowned, respected, and loved in his homeland, Einstein had to start all over again to master the skills necessary for tuberculosis work in Colorado. Even at the time of his death, at age eighty-two, he was still studying, searching into comparative religion, taking copious notes from his readings, for no other reason, said he, than "to stimulate

and deepen my mind."[22] The ideal life for Otto Einstein was total devotion to his fellow beings, no matter what the odds or
sacrifice. Over 80 percent of his Navajo patients could not understand a word he said to them but they knew instinctively
that their care was in the hands of a decent and kindly man.
"That knowledge," said Frieda Lochthowe, "led many of them
to a full and happy recovery."[23]

Aside from the handful of Navajo men admitted during the
early months of the institution's Indian health program, all of
Cragmor's Navajo patients were female. They made remarkable
progress and responded well to their enforced rest regimen as
long as the men in their lives stayed away. But once they came
under the sway of husband, brother, or sweetheart, the consumptive women, no matter how desperately ill, became the
most difficult and rebellious of patients. Some would escape by
night with their male companions, returning to the reservation
as if fleeing from prison. Others would simply go home for a
"sing," the traditional Navajo medicine dance, then suddenly
return a month or so later as though nothing unusual had tran-
spired. Their informal escapades and unannounced disappear-
ances were an unnerving element for the asylum's supervisors
and caused unproductive interruptions in their carefully pro-
grammed treatment. As long as transportation came their way,
either in the form of a man or his truck, the temptation to run
away was overwhelming; indeed, a few simply abandoned their
hospital beds and never returned.

George Dwire decided that the only solution was to eliminate
the male tempter. Hence, only female patients were admitted, visitation hours were reduced—in some cases, openly
discouraged—and the women had to be cautiously guarded
whenever their families or husbands came around. No patient
was allowed to leave the sanatorium grounds unless accompanied by a staff member. Once, however, a woman was "kid-
napped" in broad daylight by her husband and a group of his
friends who were driving through the region on a drunken
spree. It took the sheriff of Trinidad, the Colorado State Patrol,
and a carload of public health service personnel to rescue the
captive consumptive before the group could reach Raton Pass
on their way back to the mud and brush hogans of the New
Mexican desert.[24]

Once Cragmor's incarceration policy took hold, the patients were generally pleasant and cooperative. If problems arose, they were more often related to sensitive issues of lifestyle between the young girls and the older, tradition-bound women. Some of the teenagers, preferring to wear modern Anglo attire, were sternly reprimanded for any deviation from tribal customs. Other internal difficulties surfaced over religious and ritual observances. Occasionally the doctors encountered an act of stubborn refusal to be examined—the Navajo woman considered it a disgrace to undress in front of a man—or resistance to take medication. On another front, Maude Medran, the Navajo interpreter, was so fearful that the Indians would get into trouble with the lusty kitchen employees that she exacted many strict rules to insure a total Navajo segregation from the white hired help. The restrictions led to demands for her dismissal. She called the kitchen crew "white bums" and they in turn fomented contention among other employees and the Indian young people. Mrs. Medran reports that the tensions led to a near-insurrection. Finally, the authoritative voice of Annie Wauneka intervened. She not only supported Maude Medran's position, but added new restrictions of her own. Annie Wauneka's kindly but imperious presence ended all debate.[25]

And who was Annie Wauneka? Probably the single most persuasive and powerful influence on the Navajo people. In 1951 she was elected as the only woman on the Navajo Tribal Council, headquartered in Gallup, New Mexico. Shortly thereafter she became chairwoman of the Committee on Health and Welfare for the Navajo nation. Laura Gilpin depicts her as "large in stature, vigorous and strong in both mind and body, . . . a dynamic personality." She visited every hospital in the West, urging the Navajo patients to learn how to prevent contagion, accept the rest cure, and listen to the doctors' instructions. According to Gilpin, "a number of these patients, finding themselves in totally strange surroundings and among people they did not know nor to whom they could talk, became homesick and ran away. Annie brought them back, teaching them to understand the necessity of their convalescence. She helped produce a motion picture illustrating the cure and prevention of tuberculosis and acted as interpreter for the doctors and as a liaison whenever one was needed. All this was a heroic task that

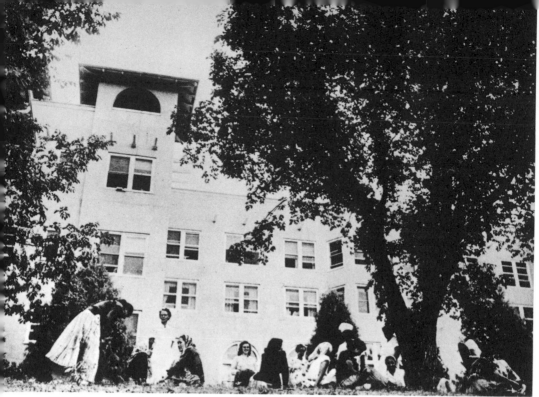

The Navajo patients at Cragmor, while all rooted in the Navajo culture, reflected the changing world in which they suddenly found themselves—some clinging to traditions and old crafts, others learning new skills and adopting modern dress.

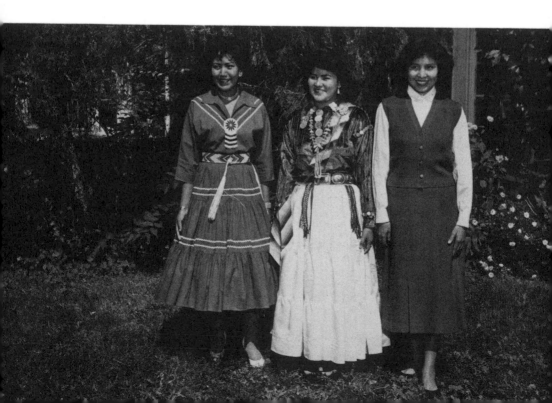

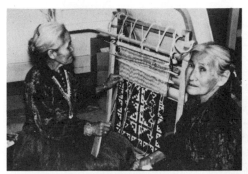

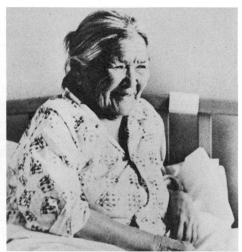

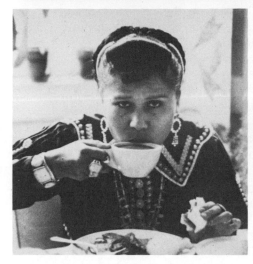

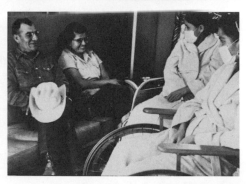

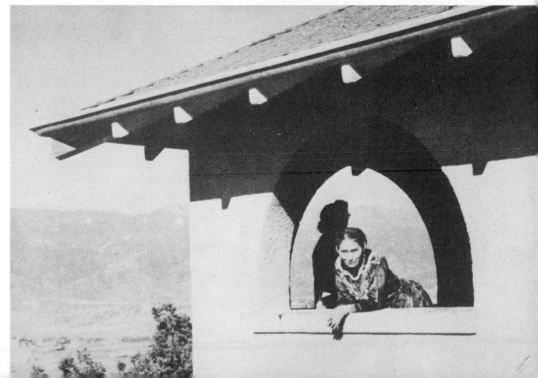

Annie pursued vigorously, using her own knowledge and persuasive powers to win these many Navajos into acceptance of
their condition and the necessity for its cure." For these achievements Annie Wauneka was one of three women named by
President John F. Kennedy to receive the Medal of Freedom.[26]

Throughout Cragmor's Indian decade, Annie Wauneka visited
the sanatorium at least twice a year. With each visit she resolved problems, instilled hope, and won the respect and ad-
miration not only of her own people but also of the doctors,
nurses, and educators at the institution.[27]

The Navajos of Cragmor ranged in age from an eight-year-old
girl to a ninety-two-year-old great-grandmother. Their conditions varied from a stage one status of chronic tuberculosis—
thus confining them to an intensive care unit and requiring as
long as six years for recovery—to a coveted stage six rating,
which allowed full mobility about the sanatorium, daily school
instruction, cooking training, and supervised visits to the super-
market, parades, picnics, elementary schools, or their favorite
haunt, the Cheyenne Mountain Zoo. A class six rating was
deemed by all to be the ideal goal. It placed them on the thresh-
old of a return to the reservation in the fullness of health.

The large population of female Navajos promoted several distinctive changes at Cragmor. In one respect they literally
changed the configuration of the floral landscape on Austins
Bluffs. Eschewing medicinal soaps and commercial shampoos,
they favored traditional Indian soap-weed, made from the yucca
root. The women made daily excursions into the bluffs, digging
up the roots of every yucca plant they could find. They would
then return to their rooms, laden with baskets of long peeled
weeds, fill their bathtubs with the natural treasure, and proceed
to chop the plants into small pieces. "We Navajos have used
country soap weeds for years," explained Margaret Platero.
"You'll live to an old age and wonder why your hair does not
turn grey. It's because Nature made the soap and it works with
the natural oils in your scalp. If you ask a Navajo why her hair
is black at the age of fifty, she will only smile. She knows you
would not believe her!"[28] Dr. Maly only shook his head with
dismay over the untouched inventory of hospital soaps and
shampoo. And later ecologists may have wondered whatever
happened to arrest the spread of Cragmor's once abundant yuc-

ca groves. The region's rich crop was all but depleted by the summer of 1954.

Another transformation at Cragmor affected the entire tradition of arts and crafts among the Navajo people. Until they entered the sanatorium, the Indian women had been adroit weavers, following the time-honored tradition of the tribe. But by the time they left the asylum, they had mastered the art of beadwork, a craft that was not native to the Navajos. So dexterous were the women in manipulating beadwork—the mainstay of Virginia Dykstra's occupational therapy program—that they invented their own geometric designs. They neither followed a predetermined model nor left any pattern for others to copy, but fashioned their own unique color schemes, creating a work of art which, according to Dykstra, soon "became an overnight sensation throughout the country."[29] The Cragmor entries at the annual Navajo Indian Fair at Window Rock won more first prizes over several successive years than were granted to any other Indian community.[30]

The patients worked day in and day out to make beaded belts, necklaces, earrings, bracelets, badges, purses, blouses, and skirts—even complete horse gear, with bridles, martingales, and leggings all intricately beaded. With repeated Navajo fair prizes, coupled with the fanfare of local exhibits and frequent news articles, their unmatched skills became widely publicized. Mail orders poured in to Cragmor from all parts of the country. People as far away as Maine and Nova Scotia requested custom-made bead necklaces. Calls and letters arrived from Houston, Oklahoma City, and Las Vegas, asking for beaded ties. Requests came from Portland, Boston, and Hollywood seeking stylish beaded quilts and jackets. Clark Gable made a special effort to secure samples of Cragmor's renowned embroidered vests and jewelry to give as gifts to his wife and friends.[31]

Soon the patients were working not simply to fill their idle hours with valuable occupational therapy but to sew, weave, and paint for commercial gain. One young woman spent six months making a beaded afghan with woven squares in subtle shades of blue and green. Another spent over a year beading a complete saddle and riding outfit. The sanatorium received over seventy cash offers for a quilt that had won a blue ribbon at the Arizona fair. Likewise, the reed and raffia baskets, crocheted rugs, quilt tops, and Indian rag dolls, all of which garnered first-place awards, caused a veritable explosion of commerical interest in the quiet sanatorium north of Colorado Springs.

Eventually George Dwire was obliged to intervene, first to check the feuding that was breaking out between a few profit-minded patients, but more importantly, to restore a balance of peace and restfulness that the outside exploitation had begun to shatter. "Cragmor will remain a curative sanatorium, not a bead factory," the talented inmates were told.[32] Yet the real problems came from the community. Dwire found it necessary to protect his protégés from the approaches of would-be entrepreneurs and craft-shop opportunists who saw a chance to exploit the patients for personal gain. More than once he had to solicit police action to chase away local pillagers and money-starved agents who had sneaked onto the grounds to appropriate the celebrated beadwork of Cragmor's congenial Navajo lungers.

One of the outstanding contributions that Cragmor made to the Indian convalescent—an offspring of Dwire's managerial foresight—was the highly successful Cragmor education curriculum. Once the Navajo's natural shyness and distrust were overcome, the women responded well to bedside and classroom instruction. The majority of the Indians came to the Anglo milieu with no understanding of English, but under such teachers as Betty Moore and Katie Veen, in a period of eighteen to twenty-four months most of them attained a third-grade level of proficiency.

Notwithstanding their rapid progress in English—along with lessons in geography, languages, algebra, typing, nursing care, and cooking—the Indians were encouraged to retain their native language. "The language barrier must never be an obstacle at Cragmor," Dwire had informed his staff. "Allow the patients to speak Navajo at every opportunity."[33] The important thing, Dwire insisted, was to preserve the Indian language to enable each woman to impart her knowledge of cooking, hygiene, and health care to her family and friends on the reservation. "Speak Navajo daily and enjoy it," Maude Medran told the women. "Never be ashamed of your beautiful Navajo ways."[34] In its own way, Cragmor inaugurated the first bilingual training school in the state of Colorado. Classroom attendance was not compulsory but nearly all of the women took advantage at some time in their cure program to learn to read and write. They then returned to the fifteen million acres of Navajo-Hopi reservation, fortified with new skills and still fluent in Navajo, eager to share their knowledge with their people.[35]

Ostensibly the Indian educational program was carried on as a positive kind of reverse psychology. Cragmor's instructors hoped to make the Navajo residents dissatisfied with their low living standards on the reservation. Mildred Dawson's cooking classes represented the strongest reinforcement of this principle. Many Navajo girls had never seen a modern kitchen before coming to Cragmor; indeed, many had never sat in a chair or eaten from a table. Dwire's intention was to expose the Indian women to progressive eating habits, instilling a respect of sanitation and proper diet, then send them back to the isolated vastness of the Southwest with a desire to impart the fundamentals they had learned about nursing care, nutrition, grooming, hygiene, and Anglo ways to their Indian companions. "The Pioneer Proselytes," Vi Murphy called them; Cragmor's own minination of Navajo converts, trained "to carry the message back to fellow Indians—better living through dissatisfaction."[36]

The Indian era brought Cragmor's long life as a care center to a fitting conclusion. Whether learning to sing Christmas carols phonetically, or sharing their arts and lifestyle with local schoolchildren, or reading Dick and Jane books to master the rudiments of English, or embroidering exquisite clothes for Hollywood celebrities, the Navajo women brought cheer, smiles, and hearty laughter to the old grey sanatorium. "They were never rude, discourteous, or surly," said Mrs. Dykstra, yet each and every individual resisted any effort to force her into a mold with which she felt incompatible. By the time Cragmor closed as a tubercular sanatorium—the last of its kind in the state—over five hundred Navajo patients had been treated, fattened on squash, fried bread, and potatoes, and returned to their hogans with an appreciation of new ways to conduct their lives.

A young Navajo named Dorothy Todacheenie summed up the experience in these simple words: "I loved my stay at Cragmor. I learned English, arithmetic, and geography. I recovered my health. I made a lot of friends. And the best part of all, I never received a scolding from anybody."[37]

SEVEN

The Last Scene of All

*When Cragmor's history ends
... I trust it will be said of us
that we did our job well.*
Alexius M. Forster

"If you do a good job you can work yourself out of employment. That is our case in helping to cure the Indians." So wrote George Dwire in a letter to U.S. Representative J. Edgar Chenoweth, expressing his dismay and bitterness over the imminent termination of Cragmor's contract with the Department of Health, Education, and Welfare.[1]

Until 1960 the sanatorium had been operating profitably as a first-class tuberculosis hospital, servicing the needs of several hundred Navajo patients. Cragmor's expenditures of some $200,000 per year provided good employment and income for many people of the Pikes Peak region. The patients arrived seriously ill and generally departed cured. The foundation's funds were sufficiently sound to permit the construction of a one-half million dollar nursing home to acommodate thirty-one aged residents. But soon afterwards the financial complexion changed. Whereas in 1958 and 1959 the state health service had increased Cragmor's number of patients to twenty-five at a time when hospitals all over Colorado were losing their tubercular wards, by 1960 the promise of sustained prosperity began to fade away. Even the gain Cragmor had hoped to secure through the closing of Glockner's tuberculosis department was not enough to pay the bills. Only twelve state patients entered the sanatorium in 1960.

George Dwire lamented the reversal of fortune with these mournful words: "During the past year, the Cragmor Foundation has had precarious times. Our number of tuberculosis patients has fallen off and the occupancy of The Manor has not advanced as rapidly as we would like. During the same period we have had many repairs to do about the grounds and buildings."[2] And later: "The number of Cragmor's patients is not sufficient to warrant the operation of a tuberculosis hospital."[3]

The most ominous threat to Cragmor's preservation came with the audit of the Indian contract, which disclosed a considerable loss of revenue. A serious misunderstanding then erupted between George Dwire and the megalithic structure of HEW. The government demanded a reimbursement of nearly $13,000 to cover discrepancies in the 1958–59 contract, while Dwire insisted that the United States Indian Service owed the Cragmor Foundation a balance of $32,000 because of a misreading of the 1959–60 agreement. The quarrel between Dwire and several federal departments continued for over eighteen months. It was a case in which George Dwire emerged victorious in battle although Cragmor lost the war. On April 15, 1961, a court decree obliged the United States Treasury to refund the sanatorium the sum of $32,233.22, as the amount owed by the United States Public Health Service for day cost of Indian patients from July 1, 1959, to June 30, 1960. But two months later, that same Public Health Service notified Dwire that the Indian contract with Cragmor was to be severed one year hence. It was a punitive and vindictive act by the government, but Dwire and the foundation could do nothing to reverse the decision. Cragmor's days were numbered. The director had twelve months in which to transfer the Navajos to Albuquerque or Tucson.

Despite several efforts to secure a sympathetic backing from state senators and representatives, Dwire saw the last of Cragmor's hopes for future funding slip away in the heat of federal strangulation. "I have been notified by telephone," he reported on December 28, 1961, "that they are going to take out the last of the Navajo patients, some eighteen in number, comprising over one-half of our patient load."[4] Six months later Cragmor surrendered its claim as one of three remaining hospitals handling Indian tuberculosis cases on a contract basis. It was judged too remote from the reservation and too small to warrant further federal assistance.[5] The commissioner of HEW informed Dwire that there was no further need for medical service to tuberculous Indians and because Cragmor's patient load had steadily declined, there was no way possible for the Public Health Service to help Cragmor's financial plight: "The economic and medical facts are catching up with us."[6]

Dwire and the foundation had no recourse but to suspend the sanatorium's operation. Ironically, its new building—the Cragmor Manor—had been dedicated only fifteen months before the institution was placed on notice that its federal support would terminate. As Cragmor closed off deserted corridors and locked its abandoned rooms, the Manor too lost its clientele. After only two years of operating as a rest home for the aged, its patients dropped off to twelve, then nine, then five, and finally to two. The last pair of Cragmor's senior citizens transferred to other local care centers in April of 1962.

The Manor was one of the region's most solidly built constructions. It was acclaimed "one of the finest institutions of its kind in the Western states," and was granted an architectural award of merit in 1961.[7] Each room in the three-story edifice boasted outside exposure, a private balcony, individually controlled heat and air conditioning, and a private or adjoining bath. Each of the sixteen apartments was equipped with an electric refrigerator, range, sink, and disposal. An audio and bell-call system connected not only the living unit but also the bathroom facilities with the nursing station on each floor. Meals were served to nonambulatory residents from the top floor dining room.

The Cragmor Manor was independent. Its elderly residents were not tuberculous. They were free to come and go as they pleased and they had nothing whatever to do with the older sanatorium area. Their building was strictly a retirement home, "a place for independence, comfort, and security."[8] Dwire considered the Manor the ideal way to meet Cragmor's changing needs in a time of declining consumptive patients. Robert Law, who served as vice-president of the Cragmor Foundation, believed it would long outlive the sanatorium proper. With words strangely reminiscent of Alexius Forster's old dictum that "there are no rules at Cragmor," Law maintained that the Manor was intended "for persons who want freedom of movement: we aren't going to put harsh rules into effect here," he said. "Nobody is happy if they have to live under harsh rules—and we want our residents to be happy."[9]

If happiness dwelt at the Manor, it was short-lived. Cragmor's attractive home for the elderly lasted for the shortest span of time among any establishment of its kind in the western United States. It was still practically new and unused when the last octogenarian was wheeled away in the spring of 1962.

What will become of Cragmor? That was George Dwire's big dilemma. As the last surviving member of the original board of directors, Dwire was looked to as the guiding oracle of wisdom and direction. And for nearly three years he pondered the problem of the empty asylum: what to do with a defunct and unfunded sanatorium in an age of widespread drug cures for tuberculosis? Cragmor was nothing but a museum piece, a dated and outworn relic of the past.

"We may turn all of our assets, amounting to some one and a half million dollars, over to the State of Colorado for free," Dwire declared in January of 1962.[10] But before giving it all away, the moribund foundation first entertained the idea of deeding several acres to El Paso County's Society for Crippled Children, an organization that saw the newly built Cragmor Manor as a possible site for physical therapy. But when the Rocky Mountain Rehabilitation Center explored the possibility of leasing or buying a portion of the property for that purpose, it found that the amount of land and the facilities were insufficient.[11]

Finally, on June 15, 1964, after several private sessions and communications with Dwire, Governor John Love authorized the University of Colorado to acquire the Cragmor property for educational purposes. Roland E. Rautenstraus, then associate dean of the faculties, met with George Dwire at President Joseph R. Smiley's behest, and negotiated the transfer of funds, endowments, and assets, identified facilities, authorized improvements, and initiated instructional and educational programs at Cragmor.[12]

During the ensuing months, the Mason C. Davidge fund was transferred to the University of Colorado as a continuous endowment. Major remodeling was undertaken at a cost of $70,000. This involved the conversion of the Solly-MacLaren sleeping porches and bedroom suites into twenty-one new classroom units; the construction of a library on the second floor of the Main Building where Cragmor once operated the finest dining hall in the Pikes Peak region; and the refurbishing of the Cragmor Manor rest home into twelve faculty offices and three administrative suites. By the late spring of 1965 the University of Colorado had engaged seven full-time faculty members in the fields of business, engineering, and political science; the Cragmor campus was ready to function.

The Colorado state legislature appropriated $25,000 for a long-range architectural study and master plan, a study that took place over the summer of 1964, prior to the opening of classes at the new Colorado Springs Center in the fall. During one of the last meetings of the Cragmor Foundation, Dean Rautenstraus stated that for all official purposes the facility once designed as the Cragmor Sanatorium would henceforth be known as the "Cragmor Campus of the University of Colorado."[13]

New generations now saunter through the labyrinthine corridors of the old Main Building, oblivious to the lessons of its sixty-year history. For most of the students, faculty, and staff of the thriving university campus the ruins on the bluff are merely ruins. The names Solly, MacLaren, and Forster are all but forgotten. The palatial dreams of Cragmor's founders, the tales of roof garden chasers, the adventures of prominent lungers, the conquests of promiscuous dandies, the unrivaled arts of the modest Navajos—all are part of the silent past. And on such a turn glides Cragmor's fate: from Edwin Solly's lovely dream to a dying lunger's last expectoration, it amounts to little more than a quiet breeze in the pines of Austins Bluffs.

NOTES

CHAPTER ONE

1. Dr. Alexius M. Forster related the following story to illustrate the common case of the "revitalized consumptive": "An old gentleman I knew came out to Colorado in 1884. When I asked him what led him to take up his residence here he said that he came with a very bad case of consumption. I told him that I supposed, of course, he had started in horseback riding on his arrival and he assured me he had. When I asked him how it worked he said that he improved very rapidly until he had a severe hemorrhage. I asked him if he went to bed following the hemorrhage and he said, 'hell, yes; I could not lift my head from the pillow for six weeks or more.' When I asked what happened next, he said that as soon as possible following the hemorrhage he got back on his horse." See "Medical Reminiscences," *Ninety-Eight-Six*, March 4, 1926, 5.

2. One of the most fascinating accounts of early migratory invalidism to the western states is Billy M. Jones, *Health-Seekers in the Southwest, 1817-1900* (Norman: University of Oklahoma Press, 1967).

3. James John Hagerman was one of the world's wealthiest men. While recovering from tuberculosis, he founded the Molly Gibson Mine near Aspen and built the Aspen extension of the Colorado Midland Railroad Company. Helen Hunt Jackson, the renowned author of *Century of Dishonor* and *Ramona*, dragged her weary frame to the Springs in 1875.

4. The origin, development, and operation of most of these health organizations are briefly described in chapter 6 of Manly D. Ormes, *The Book of Colorado Springs* (Colorado Springs: Denton Printing Company, 1933), 225–64.

5. Raymond T. Cragin, a businessman who did much to promote Cragmor and Colorado Springs in the eastern United States during the 1920s, reported that the actual cash turnover in the Springs, the year round, was due more to the health industry than to the pleasure resort. See "The Peculiar Industry of Colorado Springs," *Ninety-Eight-Six*, April 28, 1927, 1–2.

6. See Boswell P. Anderson, "What Open-Air Treatment Accomplishes in Colorado," *Colorado Springs Gazette-Telegraph*, January 1, 1905.

7. Dr. W. A. Shepard made a personal fortune building tent cottage homes beneath the willow cottonwood and balsam trees along Cheyenne Creek. He dedicated his village "to those who cough" and invited all "invalids with putrid lungs" to chase the cure in his isolated community. See *Colorado Springs Gazette-Telegraph*, May 27, 1905.

8. Letter to Edwin Solly from J. Raymond Davies, Nordrach Com-

munity, Colorado, July 18, 1905, S. Edwin Solly Papers. By the mid-1920s many responsible doctors averted panic by citing lengthy statistical studies about the low incidence of contagion from the indigent tuberculars in Colorado Springs. See, for instance, Charles Fox Gardiner, "Climate," *Ninety-Eight-Six*, February 5, 1925, 1–2; Jessamine S. Whitney, "Our Beloved Vagabonds," *Ninety-Eight-Six*, April 30, 1925, 1–3; and Henry Sewell, "Tuberculosis in Colorado," *Ninety-Eight-Six*, February 3, 1927, 1–2.

9. Information disclosed in a personal interview with Dr. H. C. Goodson, Sunnyrest Nursing Home, Colorado Springs, January 6, 1978.

10. *Mountain Sunshine*, Summer 1900, 24.

11. Letter to the editor of *Mountain Sunshine*, October 8, 1900, Solly Papers.

CHAPTER TWO

1. Undated news clipping, Solly Papers.

2. For a lively documentation of Solly's executive role during the formative years of the El Paso Club, see Marshall Sprague, "A Toast to Dr. Solly (1889–1897)," in *El Paso Club—A Century of Friendship* (Colorado Springs: El Paso Club, 1976), 13–28.

3. The Antlers had its inception on May 16, 1881, when the Colorado Springs Hotel Company was incorporated. The famous hotel opened for business June 1, 1883. See *Colorado Springs Gazette*, May 10 and June 2, 1883, and F. W. Cragin, Notebook 14, Colorado Springs Pioneers Museum.

4. This was the Town and Country course, known in later years as the Patty Jewett municipal course.

5. Jones, *Health-Seekers*, 159.

6. May 16, 1874.

7. "The Sanatorium Treatment for Tuberculosis," *Colorado Springs Gazette-Telegraph*, January 1, 1903.

8. Undated notation, Solly Papers.

9. For a concise summary of the major medical theories governing the treatment of tuberculosis in Colorado before 1900, see James H. Baker, ed., *History of Colorado*, vol. 3 (Denver: Linderman Company, 1927), 1062–64. It should not be overlooked that Dr. Henry Sewell and his wife, who had occupied one of Edward Trudeau's fresh-air cottages at Saranac Lake, New York, during the winter of 1889 also brought their impressions of the outdoor phenomenon to Colorado when they emigrated to Denver the following year. See E. L. Trudeau, *An Autobiography* (New York: Doubleday, Page and Company, 1916), 284.

10. Letter to John E. White, April 21, 1901, Solly Papers. Solly carefully distinguished his plan for a privately operated sanatorium from the more common boardinghouse convalescence familiar to Colorado

Springs invalids: "The patient will be entirely under the direction of a resident staff, where everything is regulated for him as to meals, rest, exercise, and in fact all the details of his daily life. . . . All are treated by the same doctors, upon the same principles." See *Mountain Sunshine*, Spring 1902, 28.

11. Solly served as president of the American Climatological Association, the American Laryngological, Rhinological and Onotological Society, the Colorado State Medical Society, and the El Paso County Medical Society. He also was a fellow of the Royal Medico-Chirurgical Society of London.

12. This conclusion is based on careful perusal of the Solly Papers.

13. Solly Papers.

14. The 1874 pamphlet was entitled *Manitou, Colorado, U.S.A., Its Mineral Waters and Climate*. Solly's scrapbook, containing clippings, letters, and tributes, clearly discloses the doctor's notable prestige and powers of social persuasion. He was the man who made Palmer's soda springs famous, who promoted the community better and for a longer time than anyone else had done, and who made Colorado Springs world famous as a health resort a full decade before the founding of Saranac Lake. Moreover, because of his fortuitous role as consultant in the aborted effort to erect a city-centered sanatorium, he was also the person who affected the greatest change in architectural construction of homes and medical establishments in the region. Porch, cottage, and tent designs followed the course of Solly's fresh-air doctrines. There was scarcely a home built north of town between the years 1876 and 1914, especially those in the vicinity of Colorado College, that did not in some way reflect the Solly persuasion of cottage and sleeping porch construction.

15. This was the Palmer Park portion of Austins Bluffs Park. It was officially deeded to the city by General Palmer in the winter of 1901 and was renamed Palmer Park in April of 1902. See *Facts*, April 12, 1902, 17.

16. Louis R. Ehrich, "Note," *Mountain Sunshine*, March-May 1900, 57. This is a reprint from an earlier article dated May 10, 1898.

17. Dr. White's tent community was named Nordrach Ranch. This tent city sprang into operation on November 1, 1901, only two months before General Palmer announced his gift of money and land to Edwin Solly for the development of Cragmor. White, who was also indebted to European sanatoriums for providing a model for his consumptive care center, developed a successful tent colony that in its prime (1902–1907) was the envy and prototype of every tent promoter in the country. White's success was predicated upon an undeviating insistence on outdoor survival. For a brief history of this fascinating institution, see D. R. McKay, "Chasing the Cure at Nordrach Ranch: A History of Colorado's First Sanatorium of the Open Air," *The Colorado Magazine* 56 (Winter-Spring 1979): 179–95.

18. Draft of letter, undated, Solly Papers. Compare Solly's account with the following cryptic notation that Palmer entered in his notebook

on September 30, 1901: "Promised Dr. Solly to take 50,000—3% stock or Bonds on his Austin Bluff Sanitarium to provide the ground if we could agree on location thereabouts." See William J. Palmer, 1901 Notebook, Glen Eyrie, Colorado.

19. The first board of directors, selected by William J. Palmer in consultation with Solly, included Palmer as president, Solly as vice president, J. Arthur Connell, treasurer, Gilbert McClurg, secretary, and Henry C. Hall, counsel. The five trustees were J. A. Connell, Henry C. Hall, William J. Palmer, John G. Shields, and S. Edwin Solly. The eight medical advisors consisted of Robert H. Babcock (Chicago), Samuel A. Fisk (Denver), S. A. Knopf (New York), V. Y. Bowditch (Boston), James A. Hart (Colorado Springs), Frederick I. Knight (Boston), Henry P. Loomis (New York), and James Tyson (Philadelphia). It is significant that these eastern physicians represented Cragmor's best source for securing many wealthy and influential out-of-state patients.

20. *Facts*, January 18, 1902, 3.

21. See especially the *Colorado Springs Gazette* of January 1 and 12, 1902.

22. "Freedom of Colorado Springs from Tubercular Infection," summarized in the *Colorado Springs Gazette-Telegraph*, January 19, 1902.

23. See *Colorado Springs Gazette-Telegraph*, January 19, 1902.

24. Ibid., January 12, 1902.

25. The anti-indigent campaign is described in "Our Winter Sunshine," *Colorado Springs Gazette*, January 12, 1902.

26. The second "o" in the original spelling of "Cragmoor" was dropped in April of 1902. See *Colorado Springs Gazette*, March 23, 1902, and *Facts*, March 29, 1902.

27. The editor of the *Colorado Springs Gazette*, for instance, exclaimed that this was the kind of establishment that "Colorado Springs ought to have had many years ago." March 25, 1902.

28. The release of this exorbitant figure precipitated many complaints from an unbelieving population. It led to considerable public resistance of an enterprise dubbed by one detractor in writing to Solly as "a frivolous waste of good money on bad lungs." Letter signed "Jenkins," dated April 11, 1902, Solly Papers.

29. Locally the report, containing Solly's fundamental views on sanatorium living, was reprinted in *Mountain Sunshine*, Spring 1902, 28–34. Nationally the address was disseminated in a twelve-page circular entitled "An Appeal for the Cragmor Sanatorium Association," Colorado Springs, May 1, 1902.

30. *Colorado Springs Gazette*, June 29, 1902. In contrast to these rates, the less pretentious Saranac Lake operation, founded by Trudeau many years earlier, was charging each patient only five dollars per week.

31. Account extracted from letters and clippings, Solly Papers.

32. Thomas MacLaren came to Colorado Springs as a health-seeker in 1894. Thereafter he contributed steadily to the beautification of the city. At the time Solly engaged his services, MacLaren had already designed over a dozen north end residential structures. His major accom-

plishments were still ahead of him, among them the Claremont (a residence for C. A. Baldwin, modeled after the Grand Trianon from sketches MacLaren had made at Versailles), City Hall, the Municipal Auditorium, the Burns Theatre, six churches, six schools, and several sections of the opulent Broadmoor Hotel. See Thomas Walters, *Thomas MacLaren and Colorado Springs' North End* (privately printed, n.d.).

33. The minimum size was 8 x 12 so that the sleeping porch could be used as an open-air room during the day. Adjoining the porches were bedrooms averaging 12 x 13. Between each suite MacLaren designed a bathroom to be used in common by the two neighboring occupants. The opening to the sleeping porches was to be so large that the air and sunlight would have no obstruction. The occupants could regulate the amount of sun and air admitted by means of curtains, sliding sashes, or awnings.

34. Undated memorandum to T. MacLaren, Solly Papers.

35. See "Dr. Solly Submits Cragmor Plan to Sanatorium Committee," *Colorado Springs Gazette*, February 27, 1903.

36. Glockner was established in 1890 as a home for tuberculous invalids. Its first patients paid only $7 per week, but with costs soaring everywhere about her, Mrs. Glockner, who had established the institution as a memorial to her late husband, nearly went bankrupt. To settle her debts she turned the property over to the Sisters of Charity of Cincinnati, and the hospital thereafter thrived on a benevolent and money-making plan. Ground was broken in 1902 for a surgical annex, and in April of 1903 the entire complex, known as the Glockner Sanatorium and Hospital, officially opened. For a concise summary of Glockner's early history, see Ormes, *The Book of Colorado Springs*, 233–35.

37. Communication extracted from personal letter to A. W. Fox, dated February 26, 1903, Solly Papers. Dr. John White was constantly besieged with demands to explain his quaint fresh-air methods. He insisted that "in Colorado it is absolutely possible to live out of doors every hour in the day, every day in the month and every month in the year . . . no matter what the weather is or how cold it may be." He boasted that at Nordrach he carried some twenty-five tent-living patients through one of the region's most treacherous winters when the thermometer sometimes stood at eighteen degrees below zero. See *Colorado Springs Gazette*, January 1, 1903.

38. *Colorado Springs Gazette*, February 27, 1903. One example of the mushrooming need for care facilities is seen in the hurried conversion of a downtown office building into an eighteen-room sanatorium, located at 117 North Nevada. Known as the Rocky Mountain Sanatorium, the facility operated privately, taking in all but incurable patients—from chronic consumptives to tired alcoholics seeking rest. It became so overcrowded that tents were set up in the street and in the park nearby to accommodate the overflow traffic. See *Colorado Springs Gazette*, January 1, 1903.

39. *Colorado Springs Gazette*, March 8, 1903.

40. Undated letter to Charles Markham, Solly Papers.

41. Letter to R. Bryson dated March 10, 1903, Solly Papers.

42. Letter from Elizabeth Solly to Jane Davi(d)son, dated March 23, 1903, Solly Papers.

43. Advertisements for these products may be seen in the *Colorado Springs Gazette* of April 4, 1903, and in the 1903 annual edition.

44. Quoted by Will H. Swan, "Impressions of Differences in Practice at Low and High Altitudes," *Philadelphia Medical Journal*, April 4, 1903, 7.

45. *Colorado Springs Gazette*, June 29, 1902.

46. Ibid.

47. See Samuel Edwin Solly, "Cragmor Sanatorium a Big Step Forward," *Colorado Springs Gazette*, January 31, 1904.

48. Most of Colorado Springs's winter warmth came directly from the immense coal fields of the Cragmor area. In 1904 alone, some 3,500 tons were mined daily by six companies operating in the district. At this time the south rooms of the famous Antlers Hotel were frequently filled with smoke from the electric power company's chimneys, and then, as a consequence, emptied of guests. See *Colorado Springs Telegraph*, January 31, 1904.

49. Ibid.

50. Memorandum to T. MacLaren, dated January 17, 1904, extracted from Solly Papers.

51. *Colorado Springs Gazette*, January 31, 1904.

52. Later news dispatches reported that the construction of Cragmor cost over $250,000; however, that inflated figure could only have been based on an uninformed reporter's reliance on former estimates when the Sun Palace was still on the planning board. Several years later, when Manly D. Ormes was researching material for his classic history of Colorado Springs, he wrote a letter to the superintendent of Cragmor asking for the exact cost of the original buildings. Although Laurence L. Cragin replied with a note yielding more fiction than fact, he placed "the approximate cost" of the original plant, less the Main Building and excluding equipment, at $40,420. See letter to M. D. Ormes from L. L. Cragin, December 6, 1926, Tutt Library Special Collection, Colorado College.

53. "Cragmor Sanatorium," *Colorado Springs Gazette*, December 31, 1905.

54. Extracted from a letter dated November 24, 1906, Solly Papers.

55. See the *Colorado Springs Gazette*, November 19 and 23, 1906, for Solly's obituary.

56. *Colorado Springs Gazette* editorial, November 25, 1906.

CHAPTER THREE

1. Speech notations, May 9, 1905, Solly Papers.

2. A graphic account of Palmer's accident is provided by Marshall Sprague in chapter 10 of *Newport in the Rockies* (Chicago: Swallow Press, 1971), 154–65.

3. The body whose duty it was to appoint a new medical director was the board of trustees of the Cragmor Sanatorium Association. However, the only action taken by that ineffectual organization, which at the time of Solly's death was headed by William C. Sturgis, was to issue the negative mandate to close the sanatorium "until further notice," and transfer its mischievous lungers elsewhere.

4. Henry W. Hoagland, *My Life* (Colorado Springs: privately printed, 1940), 61.

5. Ibid.

6. Ibid., 78. Overfeeding was widely practiced at Nordrach Ranch and Glockner Sanatorium. Each patient was stuffed to satiety with a rich and varied diet given in enormous quantities. The purpose of this enforced gluttony was to enable each invalid to gain between twenty-five and fifty pounds as an integral part of the cure. At Nordrach mealtime was the bedrock of Dr. White's treatment. He obliged every patient to eat twice the quantity of food desired, whether hungry or not.

7. Gardiner's frontier exploits are colorfully related by his own hand in *Doctor at Timberline* (Caldwell, Id.: Caxton Press, 1948), and by Jack Werner Schaefer in *Heroes Without Glory: Some Goodmen of the Old West* (Boston: Houghton-Mifflin Co., 1965), 253–86.

8. The Gardiner Sanitary Tent was sold and manufactured by the Colorado Springs Tent and Awning Company. Nordrach Ranch during its prime boasted seventy-two Gardiner tents. Twenty-five were erected upon the grounds of Glockner in 1903. Ten were set up near the hospital annex of the Union Printer's Home in 1904. The enterprising business was also extended over several western states and as far south as Mexico. It was later estimated, somewhat adroitly, that "fifty per cent of the patients who lived in tents recovered." That figure likewise suggests that another fifty percent succumbed—either to consumption or to nature's fury. See *Colorado Springs Gazette*, February 16, 1908.

9. Dorothy Aldridge, "Cure May Have Been Worse Than Disease," *Colorado Springs Gazette*, November 19, 1972.

10. John J. Lipset, "General Palmer: Strength in Adversity," *Colorado Springs Free Press*, March 14, 1954.

11. Information conveyed by Frieda Lochthowe, based on her personal reminiscences of conversations with Dr. Alexius Forster, successor to Drs. Hoagland, Gardiner, and Swan.

12. Letter to Mrs. Eleanor Roosevelt dated January 11, 1942. Forster received a White House reply dated January 26, 1942.

13. Forster later wrote of these experiences in two professional papers: "The Employment of Arrested Cases," *The Johns Hopkins Hospital*

Bulletin 20 (August 1909):1–14; and "The Question of Employment," *Sixth Annual Conference of the National Association for the Study and Prevention of Tuberculosis* (1910), 1–15.

14. Information conveyed by Frieda Lochthowe, based on her reminiscences of conversations with Dr. Forster. Several of these titles are among the books donated to the Colorado Springs Pioneer Museum in 1975 by Forster's daughter, Mrs. Evelyn Martin. See "Receiving Sheets," Estate of Liane Forster, August 20, 1975.

15. A. F. McKay's sojourn lasted from June 1907 through April of the following year. He boasted that he talked with every doctor east of St. Louis. The express intent of the tour was to encourage eastern physicians to send their tuberculous patients to Colorado Springs.

16. See Thomas MacLaren, "Sanatoria for Consumptives," *Brickbuilder* 17 (September 1908):177–83. The entire folio containing MacLaren's revised Sun Palace blueprints is located in the Western History Room, Pikes Peak Public Library, Colorado Springs.

17. *Colorado Springs Gazette*, September 19, 1909.

18. The influence of this executive decree led to a similar act on the national level when President Taft declared April 25, 1910, as "Tuberculosis Sunday." See *Colorado Springs Gazette*, April 25, 1910.

19. 1909 Journal, Forster Papers. The public campaign against the drinking cup was almost immediately effective. Dr. A. C. Magruder urged the city council to abolish drinking cups at the soda water springs and city fountains, recommending the substitution of sanitary fountains. The health commission supported the measure and it was approved by the council. See *Colorado Springs Gazette*, November 3 and 27, 1909.

20. 1909 Journal, Forster Papers. See also *Colorado Springs Gazette*, November 5, 1909.

21. 1909 Journal, Forster Papers.

22. Galbreath reports that such a bill was actually submitted to the Colorado state legislature in Denver. See Thomas Crawford Galbreath, *Chasing the Cure in Colorado* (University Park, 1909), 31.

23. The other individuals who bought in to Cragmor's ownership with Hayes included Benjamin Allen, called "the golden financier" by his peers; Albert E. "Bert" Carlton, the millionaire king of Cripple Creek; William A. Otis of the famed elevator clan, the same gentleman who had sold his Austins Bluffs Park estate to John White for the establishment of the Nordrach Ranch; and Clarence Carpenter, one of the city's most prominent and wealthy citizens. The combined bank holdings of these five tycoons were enough to buy every sanatorium in the state.

24. See Alexius M. Forster, "Cragmor," *Ninety-Eight-Six*, December 25, 1924, and 1910 journal notations, Forster Papers. Forster reportedly paid "upwards of $50,000 for the Cragmor." It was purchased through D. V. Donaldson of the firm of Wills, Spackman, and Kent, Colorado Springs. See "Eastern Physician Buys Cragmor," *Colorado Springs Gazette*, June 21, 1910.

25. Forster called the porch and cottage concept "the most comfortable plan of housing a tuberculosis patient," but he regarded the Gardiner Sanitary Tent as "primitive and inhuman, . . . a relic of the past, . . . a bane to comfort." He kept the tents until 1915 and used them for admission overflows and emergency lodging. See *Ninety-Eight-Six*, December 25, 1924, 1.

26. Before moving to Colorado, Forster at one time shared the view common to many physicians in the eastern United States "that the advocates of climate were a bigoted and fanatic lot, and their claims were overdrawn." Eight months of residence in Colorado completely dispelled that attitude. See A. M. Forster, "The Present Attitude toward Climate," *Proceedings of the Seventh Meeting of the National Association for the Study and Prevention of Tuberculosis* (1911), 1–23.

27. *Colorado Springs Gazette*, November 10, 1909.

28. 1910 Journal, Forster Papers.

29. Notations in 1910 and 1911 Journals, Forster Papers.

30. *Colorado Springs Gazette*, March 6 and 12, April 30, 1910.

31. Ibid., June 10, 1910.

32. Ibid., June 11 and 21, 1910.

33. Ibid., March 23, 1911. Sunnyrest, located in the Nob Hill district one mile east of the city, opened for patients on April Fools' Day, 1911. Its board of physicians included Cragmor's former codirector, Dr. H. W. Hoagland, together with Gerald B. Webb and P. O. Hanford. During its first few years of successful operation, it was managed by Sister Ida Pobschell and four other Sisters of the Kaiserwerth Deaconesses. With philanthropic assistance, Sunnyrest was the first sanatorium in the Pikes Peak region to care exclusively for the poor. It cost only $7.48 per week to support each of the seventy-seven patients handled over the first thirty months of operation. See *Colorado Springs Gazette*, October 5 and December 3, 1913.

34. Conclusions extracted from sundry notations in Forster's 1910 Journal, Forster Papers.

35. These are the very words Forster instructed T. Wynn Ross of the *Colorado Springs Gazette* to use when the incredible proposal was announced to the public on Sunday, October 6, 1912.

36. Forster's journal of 1912 contains no reference to this action. Perhaps MacLaren had good reasons of his own to walk out on Forster. Thomas MacLaren had attained a remarkably high esteem by this time. At the request of Charles A. Baldwin, he had spent a year (1906) in France studying the Grand Trianon at Versailles in order to design Baldwin's majestic "Claremont" estate. He had also designed the City Hall in Colorado Springs (1904), the public library, Elk's Home, and First Congregational Church in Boulder (1905), as well as several sumptuous Broadmoor residences.

37. In August of 1911 Barton had published a sixty-page pamphlet entitled "Preliminary Report," concerning the founding and development of the Stratton Home. Residents living near the proposed construction were enraged over the plan to build such an edifice for poor

people. They contested Winfield Scott Stratton's will and the scheme was tied up in litigation for over seven years. See Marshall Sprague, *Newport in the Rockies,* 183.

38. 1912 Journal, Forster Papers.

39. Ibid.

40. *Colorado Springs Gazette,* October 6, 1912.

41. Ibid., February 13, 1913.

42. Ibid., October 6, 1912.

43. Unsigned note to Alexius Forster, November 23, 1912, Forster Papers.

44. *Colorado Springs Gazette,* October 6, 1912.

45. Ibid.

46. 1913 Journal, Forster Papers.

47. 1911 Journal, Forster Papers.

48. The generally unheeded "Rules and Regulations" of the Cragmor Sanatorium (1911) were reprinted in *Ninety-Eight-Six,* August 5, 1926, 4, for the amusement of later sanatorium guests.

49. Information conveyed by Frieda Lochthowe.

50. In 1907 he captained the winning team in Colorado in the interstate polo tournament.

51. "Gerald Bertram Webb: Physician and Scholar" (Memorial Pamphlet), 2, Webb Memorial Library, Penrose Hospital.

52. The magazine was first called the *Cragmor News* (founded July 2, 1924), then renamed *Ninety-Eight-Six.* Webb's role in its founding was that of an encouraging godfather or patron. He urged Laurence I. Cragin and Murray P. Marcus to edit the journal. It soon became a highly regarded literary publication and lasted for seven and one-half years.

53. Marshall Sprague, "Healers in Pikes Peak History," *Denver Westerners Brand Book,* vol. 23 (Denver, 1968), 104.

54. *Overcoming Tuberculosis: An Almanac of Recovery,* coauthored with Charles T. Ryder (New York: O. B. Hoeber, 1927); *Tuberculosis* (New York: Paul B. Hoeber, 1936).

55. Webb's original research produced studies on blood morphology at high altitudes, the production of relative immunity by the gradual increase of small doses of living tubercle bacilli, the metabolism of the tubercle bacillis, and the problems of chemotherapy.

56. Sprague reports that the money for the establishment of the Colorado Foundation was put up by Alfred Cowles and other wealthy ex-Cragmorites. "This Foundation has evolved through the years into the internationally renowned Webb-Waring Institute for Medical Research at the University of Colorado Medical Center." See "Healers," 121.

57. Webb was also consulting physician to the National Methodist, Episcopal, Sunnyrest, St. Francis, and Glockner sanatoriums. He was chief of staff of Union Printer's Home from 1934 until his death.

58. Interview with George McCue, November 23, 1977.

59. Interview with Clara Jenkins, March 2, 1978.

60. *The Prescription of Literature* (Philadelphia, 1933), 1.

61. Interview with Dr. H. C. Goodson, March 17, 1978.

62. Interview with Carl Christensen, January 10, 1978.

63. *The Prescription of Literature*, 7.

64. Interview with Frieda Lochthowe, November II, 1977.

65. *The Prescription of Literature*, 11.

66. Interview with Jeannette Hilton, April 7, 1978.

67. Webb wisely feared that some books would arouse the wrong emotions among depressed tuberculars. He urged the avoidance of Anatole France, Emile Zola, Thomas Hardy, Theodore Dreiser, and Arnold Zweig. He especially counseled against Mrs. Gaskill's *Bronte Family*, which he called "the most pathetic biography ever written." The book describes in lurid detail the death of six children from phthisis.

68. Interview with Nathan Kerridge, January 12, 1978.

69. Interview with Mildred Russell, January 9, 1978.

70. Marshall Sprague, "Healers in Pikes Peak History," unpublished address, October 18, 1966.

CHAPTER FOUR

1. See *Ninety-Eight-Six*, December 25, 1924, 2.

2. Constance Pulitzer's money helped to expand the Colorado Gardens on Wood Avenue and enabled her husband, William J. Elmsley, to be president of Elton Oil Company, director of Golden Cycle, secretary of the Broadmoor Polo Association, and, after 1939, a successful rancher. In her spare time Constance served as director of the San Luis School.

3. See Don C. Seitz, *Joseph Pulitzer: His Life and Letters* (New York: AMS Press, 1924), 19–20.

4. Alexius M. Forster, "Medical Reminiscences," *Ninety-Eight-Six*, February 18, 1926, 2.

5. *Ninety-Eight-Six*, January 21, 1926, 6.

6. 1911 Journal, Forster Papers; Cragmor Sanatorium Patient Ledger, 1911–12.

7. 1912 Journal, Forster Papers; Patient Ledger, 1911–12.

8. Patient Ledger, 1911–12.

9. 1912 Journal, Forster Papers.

10. Patient Ledger, 1911–12.

11. Pneumothorax was an extremely painful procedure that involved introducing air with a needle into the pleural cavity, causing a partial collapse of the lung. Thus the diseased lung would remain at rest for a period of time. For a discussion of this treatment as practiced at Cragmor, see "Pneumothorax" by Dr. Brooks D. Good in *Ninety-Eight-Six*, September 1, 1927, 1–3. Failing this dreaded operation, Cragmor's physicians occasionally turned to the more severe practice of thoracoplasty, in which the ribs overlying the diseased portion of the lung would be removed, except for the outer covering. See B. D. Good, "Thoracoplasty," *Ninety-Eight-Six*, November 24, 1927, 1–3.

12. Patient Ledger, 1911–12.

13. 1913 Journal, Forster Papers. The incorporators included Albert E. Carlton, Alexius M. Forster, Henry C. Hall, Joel Addison Hayes, William A. Otis, Gerald B. Webb, and W. W. Williams. See "The Cragmor Sanatorium Is Incorporated," *Colorado Springs Gazette*, January 4, 1913.

14. 1913 Journal, Forster Papers.

15. *Colorado Springs Gazette*, March 24, 1914.

16. One entry in his 1914 journal echoes the earlier disillusionment: "The directors continue to dispute and rant. We have boards, hammer, and nails in hand and they take away our ladder."

17. Memorandum to A. Billing, April 27, 1914, Forster Papers.

18. *Colorado Springs Gazette*, October 4, 1914.

19. Extracted from notations, Forster Papers.

20. See Thomas Crawford Galbreath, *Tuberculosis: Playing the Lone Game Consumpion* (New York: Journal of the Outdoor Life Publishing Company, 1915), 44–54.

21. *Colorado Springs Evening Telegraph*, January 20, 1915.

22. *Ninety-Eight-Six*, April 1, 1926, 3.

23. Extracted from 1915 Journal, Forster Papers; Admission Records, 1915.

24. F. O Mathiessen, *Russell Cheney (1881–1945): A Record of His Work* (New York: Oxford University Press, 1947), 16. Cheney spent day after day assimilating Cézanne in a book of reproductions, learning about mass and structure. His desire to paint, he said, was "stronger than an unwilling body and a weak will and a sloppy brain."

25. Alexius M. Forster, "Carrie Parsell," *Ninety-Eight-Six*, August 6, 1925, 4–6.

26. Quoted in *Ninety-Eight-Six*, September 18, 1924, 2.

27. See "New Cragmor Addition to be Built upon Novel Design," *Colorado Springs Gazette*, August 17, 1919.

28. The postwar board of directors consisted of William A. Otis, president, A. E. Carlton, E. P. Shove, C. L. Tutt, W. G. Elmslie, G. B. Webb, and Alexius M. Forster.

29. Although the *Colorado Springs Gazette* of October 22, 1919, speaks of the plans having been completed, no construction actually took place.

30. Work thereon began February 20, 1920. The cost of the construction plus other remodeling amounted to $50,000. See "Biggest Building Boom in History of Springs Starts," *Colorado Springs Gazette*, February 22, 1920.

31. See A. M. Forster, "Cragmor," *Ninety-Eight-Six*, December 25, 1924, 2.

32. *Colorado Springs Gazette*, April 8 and 11, 1920.

33. "Cragmor to Extend its Scope," *Colorado Springs Gazette*, October 15, 1923.

34. *Colorado Springs Gazette*, October 21, 1923.

35. See F. M. Houck, "Industrial Convalescence," *Ninety-Eight-Six*,

September 11, 1924, 1–2; Alexius M. Forster, "The Cragmor Village Colony," *Ninety-Eight-Six*, May 28, 1925, 8.

36. Alexius Forster, "My Idea of a Sanatorium," *Ninety-Eight Six*, July 2, 1924, 1.

37. Extracted from a letter written to Frieda Lochthowe, dated September 4, 1959.

38. Interview with Henry B. Young, March 20, 1979.

39. The Cragmor Village Corporation was founded in November of 1923. Its board of directors included Drs. Frank Houck, Alexius M. Forster, and J. L. Bennett; William A. Otis of Colorado Springs; and M. Craighead of Denver.

40. Interview with Agnes H. Gray, February 8, 1978.

41. See *Ninety-Eight-Six*, May 28, 1925, 8.

42. Interview with Dora Ball, November 27, 1979.

43. Information imparted by Frieda Lochthowe.

44. Forster, "My Idea of a Sanatorium," 2.

45. W. O. Johnson, "Cragmor Rodeo a Huge Success," *Ninety-Eight-Six*, August 14, 1924, 2.

46. *Ninety-Eight-Six*, October 30, 1924, 8.

47. Some old-timers allege that McClure's less successful next novel, *Some Found Adventure* (Doubleday, 1926), was inspired by Dr. Forster's wartime romance in France. The narrative concerns an American doughboy's encounter with a young girl "with beauty, culture, and the essential charm that is French." He then dispatches her from her milieu.

48. Reid's paintings found their way to New York's Metropolitan Museum, the Corcoran and National Galleries in Washington, D.C., the Albright Gallery in Buffalo, and the Minneapolis, Detroit, and Cincinnati art museums, among others. He headed the figure painting school at the Broadmoor Art Academy from its inauguration in 1919. See Stanley Stoner, *Some Recollections of Robert Reid* (Colorado Springs: Denton Printing Co., 1934).

49. During World War II Weaver's company designed thirty-nine vital pieces of equipment for the armed forces. At his death, aged ninety-four, Weaver was considered the nation's most important inventor of modern farm implements.

50. A brief entry in the gossip column of the July 9, 1924, issue of *Ninety-Eight-Six* reads as follows: "Mr. Charles [sic] Stone of New Brighton, Staten Island, and a member of this year's class at Cornell, is the new patient in Men's Cottage 7. His mother will be with him for a while."

51. Interview with Mildred Russell, January 25, 1978.

52. 1924 Journal and notations, Forster Papers.

53. Ibid.

54. Boyd St. Clair, "A Day Will Come," *Ninety-Eight-Six*, March 5, 1925, 4.

55. "New Year Memorandum to My Staff," January 1, 1925, Forster Papers.

56. Cited in 1925 Journal, Forster Papers. Marcus was house photographer and coeditor of *Ninety-Eight-Six*.

57. Interview with Jean Buckley, November 10, 1978.

58. 1925 Journal, Forster Papers.

59. 1926 Journal, Forster Papers.

60. Among the other well-known musicians who added their talents to Cragmor's concert programs were Maria-Elise Johnson (violinist), Mary Schnitzuis Osborn (pianist), Elna Fredeen (soprano), Clara Adams (soprano), Edgar Laughlin (baritone), and Cecil Arden (mezzosoprano of the Metropolitan Opera Company).

61. See *Ninety-Eight-Six*, June 9, 1927.

62. See Clinton G. Abbott, "Cragmor Spring Bird Life," *Ninety-Eight-Six*, July 4, 1929, 1–3.

63. Interview dated January 18, 1979.

64. Letter from Boyd St. Clair, St. Louis, Missouri, August 18, 1925, Forster Papers.

65. The Little Shop first opened in September of 1926. It lasted for almost five years. At times it was used as an art gallery. George Elbert Burr displayed his etchings of the American desert there and Laura Gilpin sold several of her photographs of the area.

66. Interview dated January 20, 1978.

67. Information conveyed by Harry English, collector, Falls Church, Virginia.

68. *Ninety-Eight-Six*, July 9, 1925, 10.

69. Ibid.

70. This edifice was intended originally for patients. Later, following the disastrous collapse of the nurses' home on the bluff behind the Main Building and a sudden decline in patients during the early 1930s, the new building became a second refuge for Cragmor's displaced nurses. Its construction is described in the *Colorado Springs Gazette*, May 14, 1927, and in *Ninety-Eight-Six*, May 26, 1927, 9. More than fifty years after its construction, an enterprising name campaign conducted by the faculty of the University of Colorado at Colorado Springs still failed to confer a title to this name-deprived building, except to call it by the unimaginative and obvious appellation of South Hall.

71. Information provided by L. L. Cragin in correspondence with Manly D. Ormes, December 6 and 10, 1926, and February 26, 1927.

72. At that time, according to Dr. Forster's journal notations, there were only 70,000 sanatorium beds in the United States. Medical reports estimated that of the country's one million consumptives, one tenth of them, or 100,000 persons, died each year. 1927 Journal, Forster Papers.

73. Raymond T. Cragin, "The Peculiar Industry of Colorado Springs," *Ninety-Eight-Six*, April 28, 1927, 1–2.

74. Chase Stone rented everything from a one-engine biplane, charging one penny a pound, to a three-engine Bach. In February of 1930 the large aircraft transported sightseers over Pikes Peak for $17.50.

75. The sun cure for consumption originated when a doctor observed how the peasants in the Swiss Alps cured their meat by exposing it to

the sun. He decided to try the method on wounds, and observed the excellent results in tuberculous ulcers. Cragmor's special application of heliotherapy is best documented in the following accounts: Murray P. Marcus, "Heliotheraping at Rollier," *Ninety-Eight-Six*, July 9, 1924, 2–3; Charles E. Sevier, "The Sun God's Cure," in four parts, *Ninety-Eight-Six*, from March 18 to May 13, 1926; a pamphlet entitled *The Sun Cure at Cragmor* (Cragmor Sanatorium, 1926); and Gerald B. Webb's engaging articles, "Heliology and Heliosis," in seventeen parts, *Ninety-Eight-Six*, from October 29, 1925, to February 3, 1927. These latter publications constitute a series of literary essays on the evolution of "sunrayism."

76. Notations, 1911 Journal, Forster Papers.

77. Dr. Sevier, born in Tennessee in 1889, was another among Cragmor's physicians who came to Colorado on account of ill health. He spent two years (1922–23) chasing the cure, then became a member of the institution's staff in 1926.

78. Information conveyed by Frieda Lochthowe.

79. See Ishbel MacLeish, "Half-Way House," *Ninety-Eight-Six*, September 16, 1926, 7–8, and "Half-Way House: A Curative Workshop," *Ninety-Eight-Six*, September 27, 1928, 3–4. Half-Way House was established by Ishbel MacLeish and Sophie B. Morris of Cragmor in league with May Howbert and Margaret Anderson. Oscar Magnuson was hired as occupational therapist. The shop opened at 832 North Cascade Avenue in the large dwelling that was once the Grace Church Parish House. On October 1, 1926, it moved to 27 East Platte Avenue, opposite the El Paso Club. Again in September of 1928 it made its final move, to 12 East Boulder Street. There it evolved from a private enterprise into a Community Chest agency. See "Half-Way House Annual Report," October 1956; and Gudrun T. Sack, "The Half-Way House," *Ent-ries*, 6 (October 1956) (ENT Air Force Base Publications), 1, 6–7.

80. Quoted in *Ninety-Eight-Six*, January 30, 1930, 5.

81. "Cragmor Magazine Is One of Best in the West Now," *Colorado Springs Gazette*, May 3, 1925.

82. Ellingson served on the staff of the *Colorado Springs Gazette* from 1923 until his death in 1952. For a summary of the journal's early history see *Ninety-Eight-Six*, June 19, 1930, 8–9.

83. Ashley's essay on American novelists deals with Hemingway, Christopher Morley, and Willa Cather. See *Ninety-Eight-Six*, February 4, 1926.

84. See, for example, the January 7, 1926, special poetry issue of *Ninety-Eight-Six*, wherein several of the eighteen reprinted poems, edited by Henry Harrison of the New York Circle of Bookfellows, were written by Cragmorites. Also see "A Potpourri of Poetry and Verse," *Ninety-Eight-Six*, July 8, 1926, 2–9.

85. See Sudie E. Pyatt, "Whither the Tuberculosis Periodical?" in *The Journal of the Outdoor Life*, February 1929, reprinted in *Ninety-Eight-Six*, February 14, 1929, 7–10. One prominent gentleman selected Cragmor over other sanatoriums because of its journal's fine reputation. Eugene

Lilly came in December of 1925 and chased the cure at Cragmor for more than two years.

86. Interview with Elizabeth Gunnison, March 11, 1979.

87. W. H. B., "Concerning Colorado Birds," *Ninety-Eight-Six*, December 11, 1924, 4.

88. Mrs. Low's two-part study about Cragmor's birds is appropriately entitled "Our Feathered Friends." See *Ninety-Eight-Six*, January 20 and February 17, 1927.

89. Abbott's published observations are "Wild Life at Cragmor," *Ninety-Eight-Six*, February 28, 1929, 1–3; "Cragmor's Spring Bird Life," *Ninety-Eight-Six*, July 4, 1929, 1–3; and "From Field and Study," *San Diego Society of Natural History* 31 (February 15, 1929) :124–25.

90. Papetown was located in that area now populated by the industrial and commercial world of Fillmore Street, between Hancock Street and North Nevada Avenue.

91. The same may be said for the infamous racketeer "Lucky" Luciano, who allegedly derived more money than pleasure operating a casino at the old William Otis manor off Chelton Road, the same site once occupied by the Nordrach Ranch Sanatorium.

CHAPTER FIVE

1. Sprague, "Healers," 120.

2. *Ninety-Eight-Six*, July 19, 1928, 14.

3. 1928 Journal, Forster Papers.

4. Unsigned note dated July 13, 1930, Forster Papers.

5. One such show was the staging of a major theater production on Thanksgiving Day in 1930. Local talent prepared a three-act comedy entitled *The Patsy*, directed by Cragmorite Julio Averill and performed "in the grand manner" with footlights, drapes, and an elaborate stage setting on the dining hall. It was the last large-scale cultural event in Cragmor's history.

6. February 1930 announcement to all Cragmor guests, Forster Papers.

7. Announcement to all Cragmor guests, April 15, 1930, Forster Papers.

8. Interview with George McCue, November 23, 1977.

9. Ibid.

10. Interview with Frieda Lochthowe, August 8, 1978.

11. Unsigned complaint dated April 1930, Forster Papers.

12. See B. C. D., "Cragmor Impressions," *Ninety-Eight-Six*, July 18, 1929, 8.

13. Ibid.

14. 1929 Journal, Forster Papers.

15. *Ninety-Eight-Six*, May 12, 1927, 1.

16. See M. L. T., "In Favor on Ninety-Eight-Six," *Ninety-Eight-Six*,

November 7, 1929, 4, and R. D. Whittemore's article, "Hold Your Horses," which lampoons the sporadic outbursts of rebellion on the part of puritanical readers, in *Ninety-Eight-Six*, November 21, 1929, 1.

17. 1929 Journal, Forster Papers.

18. Shortly before his death, Jim Webb wrote three installments for *Ninety-Eight-Six* on the Old West concerning his former days in the Colorado mining camps when "crude times bred crude events." See "Just a Few Years Ago," *Ninety-Eight-Six*, June 10, 1926, 1–3; August 5, 1926, 7–9; and August 19, 1926, 7–8.

19. Ibid., February 2, 1928, 10; March 15, 1928, 6.

20. Part of the costs were subsidized through benevolent gifts from W. R. Coe of New York and Spencer Penrose and A. E. Carlton of Colorado Springs. See *Colorado Springs Gazette*, July 13, 1930, and *Ninety-Eight-Six*, September 12, 1929, 12.

21. See *Colorado Springs Gazette*, May 30, 1931.

22. Ibid., November 24, 1935.

23. The FERA was a government forerunner of the welfare plan, set up to provide relief for families needing food, shelter, clothing, and medical care. It serviced the needs of 23,000 Colorado families receiving unemployment relief in 1933. The agency was liquidated in 1937.

24. Robert Rhea had first entered Cragmor in 1912, suffering from chronic pulmonary tuberculosis. He returned again in 1914, the victim of frequent hemorrhaging. After the world war he was readmitted a third time, having experienced a relapse of consumption with complications of influenza and pneumonia. That he ever survived was, in Dr. Forster's words, "one of God's unspoken miracles." Rhea, like Chase Stone, rose to prominence in local business concerns. See 1936 Journal, Forster Papers.

25. *Colorado Springs Gazette-Telegraph*, February 16, 1936.

26. Ibid.

27. Andrés Herrera's three Cragmor diaries were bequeathed to Frieda Lochthowe.

28. The foundation had its laboratories in Palmer Hall of Colorado College. It became one of the leading nonprofit tubercular research centers in the country. By 1937 it had achieved an endowment fund of $161,000. Experimenting with monkeys, the foundation completed studies on the extraction of active substances from the tubercle bacilli, the efficacy of certain vaccinations, and the effect of solar radiation on the death rate from tuberculosis. Eight major publications resulted from the Colorado foundation's research. See Gerald B. Webb, "The Colorado Foundation for Research in Tuberculosis," *Ninety-Eight-Six*, February 5, 1925, 6; August 13, 1928, 1; and "Monkey Experiments," *Colorado Springs Gazette*, October 10, 1937.

29. Interview with George McCue, November 27, 1977.

30. Interview with Maxine H. Sain, February 17, 1978.

31. See "Sanatoriosis," *Ninety-Eight-Six*, October 22, 1931, 4; and interview with Preston Sumner, February 8, 1978.

32. Notation dated January 1931, Forster Papers; see also *Colorado Springs Gazette*, January 5, 1931.

33. Interview with Sarah Mae Winford, May 3, 1978.

34. Interview with Jerald Morrison, March 9, 1978.

35. Interview with Frieda Lochthowe, December 17, 1977.

36. "Announcement to Guests" (1935), Forster Papers.

37. Chase Stone Papers, courtesy Mead Stone of McGraw-Hill, Inc.

38. Interview with Frieda Lochthowe, April 20, 1978.

39. Ibid.

40. Ibid.

41. Forster loaned the Cragmor Foundation $7,252.24 on a two-year promissory note. However, because the foundation ran into hard times, Forster was not fully repaid until April of 1939. At that first meeting of the Cragmor Foundation (March 31, 1936), Alexius M. Forster was elected president and managing editor; Perry Greiner, vice-president; Philip Jankowitz, secretary-treasurer; and H. T. McGarry, assistant treasurer. Greiner resigned in October and was replaced by George J. Dwire. Jankowitz, who angrily protested that certain illegalities in the transition from Cragmor's private ownership to its nonprofit status had left him bereft of much personal property, resigned his post in a huff in January of 1937, following which Dwire became the new secretary and treasurer of the foundation and Dr. Brooks D. Good was elected vice-president. See "Minutes of the Board of Directors," *Record of Proceedings* 1 (July 31-October 28, 1938), 2–23; April 21, 1939), 45–46.

42. See *Record of Proceedings* 1 (December 15, 1937), 31–35.

43. The so-called New Building was empty and unused at this time, as were the garage, the greenhouse, and the laundry. See *Record of Proceedings* 1 (December 28, 1938), 40.

44. Interview of January 25, 1978.

45. Interviews with Cragmor's former employees and patients about practices during this period, in contrast with the fun-loving and generally laudatory and favorable comments made in earlier chapters, resulted in many negative and under-the-table disclosures. Many informants insisted on anonymity in return. Thus, those who supplied information about conditions, personalities, practices, etc., during this troubled era in Cragmor's history are left unidentified.

46. The illegal practice took place on the ground floor of the Main Building in a room marked No Admittance. One aide reports that a condition of her being hired "was to mind my own business. . . . When there were operations being performed, we were not allowed near the operating table. . . . All the bandages and other questionable items were burned over the bluff away from the hospital." One former nurse has reported that "over one hundred abortions may have taken place at Cragmor" over a seven-year period.

47. The foundation's attorney, H. T. McGarry, requested the meeting and insisted that the minutes had to include an explicit denial of the board's awareness of any previous abortions at Cragmor, together with

a strong disapproval of the practice. See *Record of Proceedings* 2 (September 22, 1947), 65.

48. Ibid.

49. See "Contract for the Care and Treatment of Tuberculous Patients at Cragmor Sanatorium," an agreement executed April 19, 1943, in Cleveland, Ohio, between the medical staff of Cragmor and the Grand Lodge of the Brotherhood of Railroad Trainmen.

50. These buildings represented an investment of $85,000. The two boilers in the power plant, plus most of the copper and brass equipment in both edifices, were sold to the United States Air Force Base at Salina, Kansas. See "Two Buildings at Cragmor Razed," *Colorado Springs Gazette-Telegraph*, November 15, 1942.

51. *Record of Proceedings* 2 (June 17, 1942), 52.

52. Ibid.

53. Ibid., September 4, 1946, 63.

54. Unlike the Cleveland railroad men before them, Cragmor's veterans were all comsumptives. Excepting a very few who were actually bedridden, they were generally hearty individuals, much more ambulant than the resident civilian patients.

55. See "Opposes Removing Vets from Cragmor," *Colorado Springs Free Press*, August 27, 1947.

56. This image, a regrettable contrast to the Forster of earlier days, was compiled from numerous interviews.

57. *Record of Proceedings* 2 (November 3, 1947), 66.

58. Ibid., March 10, 1948, 68.

59. Ibid., April 26, 1948, 72.

60. Mrs. Coxwell was a widow from Mobile, Alabama. She had come to Cragmor following her husband's death in the 1918 influenza epidemic. She and Forster were close friends for over thirty years.

61. Letter from E. James Brady, M.D., clinical director, to the Cragmor Foundation board of directors, January 24, 1953.

62. *Record of Proceedings* 2 (September 23, 1954), 93–94.

CHAPTER SIX

1. Information concerning Yosemite Nabona is based on an unpublished essay and miscellaneous notations collected by Carl Hogue, a Cragmor Navajo and editor of *Cragmor: Corn of the Rainbow* (1953–59). Material provided courtesy of Frieda Lochthowe.

2. See "The Indian Doctor," *Ninety-Eight-Six*, January 31, 1929, 9.

3. Interview with Dolores Brown, May 3, 1978.

4. Correspondence with John Norris, January 18, 1978.

5. See *Record of Proceedings* 2 (September 10, 1953), 89.

6. Note to G. Dwire dated February 3, 1956, Dwire Papers, courtesy Agnes Dwire.

7. During one year's time the foundation's assets increased by

$77,203. Expenditures for repairs and improvements amounted to $47,500 in 1955 and $105,000 the following year. It was George Dwire's intention to beautify the grounds as he remembered seeing them thirty years earlier. See *Record of Proceedings* 3 (February 1, 1955), 1; (February 1, 1956), 11–12.

8. The major improvements included the construction of a sewage disposal field (1953–54), fire walls (1955), a new roof on the Main Building (1955), the installation of a new water main (1956), and the revamping of the Old Home Cottage (1956). See *Proceedings* 3, 1–14.

9. Ibid., 21.

10. From handwritten notes to a speech by George Dwire, ca. 1955.

11. Letter from James R. Shaw, M.D., Arizona Medical Center, Tucson, Arizona, May 23, 1978.

12. Anonymous disclosures.

13. Interview with Dr. Lewis A. Crawford, January 6, 1978.

14. Ibid.

15. Letter from Shaw, May 23, 1978.

16. Interview with Florence Ingraham, April 18, 1979.

17. Interview with Frieda Lochthowe, November 21, 1978.

18. Interview with Annie May Anderson, January 28, 1978.

19. Extracted from Einstein funeral oration, given by Rabbi Kaiman, February 1959.

20. Interview with Frieda Lochthowe, November 21, 1978.

21. Interview with Maxine H. Sain, February 5, 1978.

22. Einstein funeral oration, February 1959.

23. For information on Dr. Otto Einstein, see *Cragmor: Corn of the Rainbow*, 6; *Record of Proceedings* 3, 26, with attached Resolution, "Eulogy for Dr. Otto Einstein," by Rabbi Arnold G. Kaiman, Colorado Springs Jewish Synagogue; obituary notice, *Colorado Springs Gazette*, February 9, 1959; Einstein papers, courtesy Einstein family and Frieda Lochthowe.

24. Information provided by Frieda Lochthowe.

25. Interview with Maude Medran, May 15, 1978.

26. Laura Gilpin, *The Enduring Navajo* (Austin: University of Texas Press, 1968), 169. With the establishment in 1955 of the United States Public Health Service, which assumed the work of the Department of Health of the Bureau of Indian Affairs, Councilwoman Wauneka's role became one of interpretation and communication. She won her people's cooperation by visiting all of the contract hospitals and sanatoriums in the western states, persuading ill Navajos to accept the government-sponsored medical program.

27. An example of Annie Wauneka's forceful influence at Cragmor is documented by Margaret Platero, an Indian patient, in "Navajo Councilwoman's Visit," *Cragmor: Corn of the Rainbow* 10 (July-August 1954): 2–3.

28. Platero's recipe for a home-brewed yucca plant shampoo is printed in *Cragmor: Corn of the Rainbow* 9 (June 1954) :1.

29. Interview with Virginia Dykstra, February 1, 1978.

30. In 1957, for instance, Cragmor won twenty-eight prizes at the eleventh annual Navajo fair, a record in its time. See Mildred Meeker, "Navajo Arts Flourish at Cragmor Here," *Colorado Springs Free Press,* October 20, 1957.

31. This and subsequent information about Cragmor Navajo crafts conveyed by Mildred Dawson, Virginia Dykstra, and Betty B. Moore.

32. Quoted by Frieda Lochthowe.

33. Interview with Katie Veen, January 10, 1978.

34. Interview with Maude Medran, May 15, 1978.

35. See "Hospitalized Navajo-Hopi Maidens Gain Health, Skills at Cragmor," *Colorado Springs Free Press,* May 7, 1957; and "Navajo Sanatorium Public Schools," *Denver Post,* March 24, 1957.

36. Vi Murphy, "Navajo Patients Learn How to Raise Living Standards," *Colorado Springs Gazette,* March 2, 1958.

37. From Carl Hogue, notations for *Cragmor: Corn of the Rainbow,* courtesy Frieda Lochthowe.

CHAPTER SEVEN

1. Letter dated January 17, 1962, from George J. Dwire, D.D.S., to the Honorable J. Edgar Chenoweth, Washington, D.C.

2. Report to the Board of Directors by George J. Dwire, managing director, January 16, 1961.

3. Letter to John A. Carroll, United States Senate, from George J. Dwire, December 29, 1961.

4. Letter to W. L. Mitchell, Department of Health, Education, and Welfare, Washington, D.C., December 28, 1961.

5. Cragmor's closing statistics indicated an average of sixteen patients registered in 1960 and eighteen in 1961.

6. Letter to George J. Dwire from W. L. Mitchell, January 4, 1962.

7. See *Colorado Springs Gazette,* February 28, 1960, and September 16, 1961.

8. Ibid.

9. *Colorado Springs Free Press,* February 28, 1960.

10. Letter to John A. Carroll, United States Senate, January 17, 1962.

11. *Colorado Springs Gazette,* June 29, 1962; see *Record of Proceedings* 3 (February 21, 1963), 71.

12. See correspondence of J. R. Smiley and R. C. Rautenstraus with George J. Dwire, June 16 and 24, 1964; *Record of Proceedings* 3 (June 11, 1964), 86; letter from Robert Dunlap, attorney at law, to the board of directors, Cragmor Foundation, Inc., dated July 15, 1964.

13. See *Record of Proceedings* 3 (May 26, 1965), 92–93. For a record of the early history of the Colorado Springs Extension Division and campus activities at the Cragmor site, see Helen T. Foster, "The Origins of the University of Colorado at Colorado Springs, 1952–1975," unpublished master's thesis, Department of History, UCCS, 1976.

ACKNOWLEDGMENTS

For resource materials used in the preparation of this book, I am indebted to Dr. George V. Fagan, Head Librarian, and his capable staff in Special Collections at the Charles Leaming Tutt Library, Colorado Springs; Ms. Nancy Loe, Local History Librarian, Western History Department, and her competent assistants at the Pikes Peak Regional Library of Colorado Springs; and Mrs. Rosemary Hetzler of the Pioneers' Museum, Colorado Springs. Appreciation is also expressed to Dr. Michael Herbison, Director of the Library, University of Colorado at Colorado Springs, for his unfailing assistance and encouragement. Other institutions and agencies that have likewise accorded time and facilities to lighten the burden of research include the University of Colorado Medical Center, the Western History Department of the Denver Public Library, the Social Science and History Division of the Chicago Public Library, the Colorado Springs Chamber of Commerce, the American Medical Association, and the El Paso County Medical Society. A words of thanks also to Connie Gelvin of the Colorado Springs chapter of the American Lung Association, Margaret Butts, formerly of the Denver chapter of that organization, and Dr. Carl W. Tempel of the Jewish Consumptive Relief Federation. My appreciation as well to Sister Dolores, Assistant Librarian of the Webb Memorial Library of Colorado Springs, and Dr. Ronald A. Nelson of Fitzsimons Army Medical Center of Denver.

To the many individuals who either consented to be interviewed or corresponded from afar, I owe a heartfelt expression of gratitude. It is singularly difficult to name all willing contributors, risking the possibility of an occasional omission. But I would be most ungrateful not to mention the splendid help accorded me by the following people, and I trust that those who find their names missing from this alphabetical listing will know that they have my warmest personal thanks for their help: Annie May Anderson; Dr. Catherine Anthony of Denver; Dora and Roy Ball; Azalea Barley; Dr. Harry Basehart of the Department of Anthropology, University of New Mexico; Maude Boulton; Rhea N. Boyden; Rita Brickley; Jean Buckley; Gladys Bueler; Glynda Carpenter; Carl and Emma Christensen; Dr. Lewis A. Crawford; Jonathan Davies; Mildred Dawson; Dr. Kurt W. Deuschle of the Mount Sinai School of Medicine; Josianne Forster Doyle of Phoenix, Arizona; Robert Dunlap; Agnes Dwire; Virginia Dykstra; Dr. Robert Einstein of Beverly Hills, California; Harry English of Falls Church, Virginia; Major M. Fennell; Tony Fontana; Elaine Freed; Miles Garner; Mrs. G. B. Gilbert; Laura Gilpin of Santa Fe, New Mexico; Blanche Glynn; Dr. H. C. Goodson; Agnes H. Gray; Elizabeth Gunnison; Jeannette Hilton; Glenn Hutchinson; Florence Ingraham; Mrs. Horace R. Iverson, M.T. Jarman of Cleveland, Ohio; Clara Jenkins; Robert H. Johnson; Nathan Kerridge; Naomi Kuhlman; Marian Lewis; Eugene Lilly; Frieda Lochthowe, who gave me many hours of her time and access to extremely valuable materials; Rose Lorig; George McCue; Dr. Walsh McDermitt; Mrs. John L. McDonald; Evelyn Forster Martin; Vernie Martz; Maude Medran; Betty B. Moore; Jenny Morris; Jerald Morrison; Mrs. Aidan M. Mullett; Barbara Norris of Philadelphia; Phillip B. Owens of Los Angeles; Betty Paige; Juan Reid; Evelyn S. Ross; Mildred Russell; Maxine H. Sain; C. Saleny; Floyd Sellers; Dr. James R. Shaw of the Arizona Medical Center, Tucson; Hestor and Mittie Sircy; Marion Sondermann; Marshall Sprague; Helen Starkey; Mrs. John W. Stewart; Mead Stone; Mrs. A. J. Stubblefield of Seattle; Preston Sumner; W. A. Swanberg of Newton, Connecticut; Minnie Teague; Gussie Templeton; Lew Tilley; John Tolliver; Katie Veen; Tony Venetucci; Thomas Walters of Denver; Florence Warner; Annie Wauneka of Window Rock, Arizona; George M. Wilson; Margaret Wilson of Englewood, Colorado; Sarah Mae Winford; Mrs. Fred Wolf; Henry B. Young; and Mrs. Daniel Zuniga.

Several of these individuals donated photographs, pamphlets, scrapbooks, diaries, clippings, letters, and miscellaneous documents, and granted permission for the reduplication of family photos and other materials that I have used in this book or in special exhibits and slide lecture programs. I am most appreciative of their generous assistance. Cloyd and Dan Brunson of Stewarts Commercial Photography, Colorado Springs, deserve recognition for their sensitive care in restoring and reproducing the old photographs.

A project of this magnitude will tend to reopen old wounds, just as it rekindles fond memories. To those people who, for whatever reason, chose to divulge information about Cragmor with the proviso that I honor their anonymity, I take this opportunity to thank them, one and all, for their useful assistance, and to pledge my ongoing respect for the confidentiality of their reporting.

The University of Colorado community deserves commendation for its valued encouragement and financial support. In this connection I wish to acknowledge the help of former President Roland C. Rautenstraus, Dean James A. Null, Professor José B. Fernández, now of Orlando, Florida, and Mr. Thomas McLaughlin for their able and kind assistance.

My colleagues and friends who so kindly gave of their time to read the manuscript and to offer critical suggestions in the task of revision include Alexander Blackburn, Bruce Buck, Tom McLaughlin, Hastings Moore, and Marshall Sprague. I am particularly grateful to Marshall for his gracious willingness to write a brief Foreword to this book; I deem it a distinct honor to accept this act of kindness from a fine scholar and superb human being.

I express appreciation to Cathryne Johnson, Judy Gamble, and the Publications Department staff of the Colorado Historical Society for their perceptive editing and helpful suggestions.

BIBLIOGRAPHY

PUBLISHED SOURCES

Barton, George Edward. *Preliminary Report: An Analysis of the Conditions Influencing the Building of the Myron Stratton Home and Recommendations for Its Foundation and Development* (pamphlet). Colorado Springs, August 1911.

Benevolent Institutions. Washington, D.C.: United States Department of Commerce, Bureau of the Census, 1910.

Buckman, George Rex. *Colorado Springs and Its Famous Scenic Environs.* 2d ed. Colorado Springs, 1893.

The Campaign of the Modern Woodmen of America Against Tuberculosis (pamphlet). Woodmen Press, 1909.

Chapman, Arthur. *The Story of Colorado.* Chicago: Rand McNally, 1924.

Colorado Souvenir Book for the International Congress on Tuberculosis. Denver: Colorado State Organization, 1908.

Colorado Springs Evening Telegraph.

Colorado Springs Free Press.

Colorado Springs Gazette.

The Colorado Springs Region as a Health and Pleasure Resort. 4th ed. Colorado Springs: Chamber of Commerce, 1903.

Cragmor (pamphlet). Colorado Springs: Cragmor Sanatorium, 1926.

Cragmor: Corn of the Rainbow. Edited by Carl Hogue. Sanatorium newsletter published irregularly by the Navajo patients, 1953–59.

Cragmor Hurricane. Colorado Springs: Cragmor Sanatorium. Volume 1 began in January 1950.

Cragmor News. Colorado Springs: Cragmor Sanatorium. Volume 1 began with issues dated 1949.

Cragmor Sanatorium for the Treatment of Tuberculosis (pamphlet). Colorado Springs: Out West Printing and Stationery Company, 1905.

Denison, Charles. *Rocky Mountain Health Resorts: An Analytic Study of High Altitudes in the Arrest of Chronic Pulmonary Disease.* Boston: Houghton, Osgood, and Company, 1880.

————. "The Sleeping Canopy." *Transactions of the American Climatological Association* 28 (1907).

Directory of Colorado Springs and Manitou. Colorado Springs: R. L. Polk and Company, 1911–1948.

Directory of Sanatoria. New York: Livingston Press, 1931.

Dunbar, Simeon J., Mrs. *The Health Resorts of Colorado Springs and Manitou.* Colorado Springs: Gazette Publishing Company, 1883.

Elder, Charles S. "Medicine." In *History of Colorado*, edited by James H. Baker vol. 3. Denver: Linderman Company, 1927.

Facts. Colorado Springs: Facts Publishing Company, 1900–1901.

Forster, Alexius M. "The Employment of Arrested Cases." *Johns Hop-*

kins Hospital Bulletin 20 (August 1909): 1–14.

————. "The Present Attitude Toward Climate." In *Transactions.* Seventh Annual Meeting of the National Association for the Study and Prevention of Tuberculosis, 1911.

————. "The Question of Employment." In *Transactions.* Sixth Annual Meeting of the National Association for the Study and Prevention of Tuberculosis, 1910.

Frost, R. E. *Beloved Professor.* New York: Vantage Press, 1961.

————. "The Fallible Dr. Robert Koch." *Journal of American Medical Association* 198 (December 26, 1966): 111.

Galbreath, Thomas Crawford. *Chasing the Cure in Colorado.* Privately printed, 1909.

————. *TB: Playing the Lone Game Consumption.* New York: Journal of the Outdoor Life Publishing Company, 1915.

Gardiner, Charles Fox. *The Care of the Consumptive.* New York: G. P. Putnam's Sons, 1900.

————. *Climate of Colorado Springs: Its Therapeutic Value in Treating TB.* Reprinted as *The Therapeutic Gazette.* Colorado Springs, 1926.

————. *The Colorado Springs Region as a Health Resort: High Altitudes for Invalids.* Colorado Springs Chamber of Commerce, 1898.

————. *Doctor at Timberline.* Caldwell, Id.: Caxton Printers, 1938.

————. "The Importance of an Early and Radical Climate Change in the Case of Pulmonary Tuberculosis." *New York Medical Journal* (August 24, 1901).

————. "Light and Air in the Treatment of Consumption in Colorado." *Medical News* (July 22, 1899).

————. "The Sanitary Tent and Its Use in the Treatment of Pulmonary Tuberculosis." *Transactions of the American Climatological Association* 18 (1902).

Gardner, S. A. "A Trip to Colorado in 1878." *Peoria Evening Call* (July 27, 1878).

Gilbert, G. Burton. "G. B. Webb," *Transactions of the American Clinical and Climatological Association* 60 (1948).

The Glockner Sanatorium (pamphlet). Colorado Springs: Glockner Sanatorium Press, ca. 1912.

Hafen, LeRoy R., ed. *Colorado and Its People: A Narrative and Topical History of the Centennial State.* Vol. 2. New York: Lewis Historical Publishing Company, 1948.

Half-Way House Annual Report (pamphlet). Colorado Springs: Half-Way House; October 1956.

Hannemann, Judith. "Four Physicians and Their Bookplates." *University of Colorado Quarterly* 11 (Fall 1969): 4-10.

Hart, James A. "In Memoriam: Samuel Edwin Solly, M.D., M.R.C.S." *Transactions of the American Climatological Association* 23 (1907).

Hilton, Emeline L. J. *The White Plague.* Duluth, Minn.: M. I. Stewart Company, 1913.

Hoagland, Henry Williamson. *My Life.* Colorado Springs: Privately printed, 1940.

Howbert, Irving. *Memories of a Lifetime in the Pikes Peak Region*. Putnam, 1925.

Jones, Billy M. *Health-Seekers in the Southwest, 1817-1900*. Norman: University of Oklahoma Press, 1967.

Journal of Outdoor Life. New York: The National Tuberculosis Association. Various issues, 1920s and 1930s.

Kitch, John I. *Woodmen Valley: Stage Stop to Suburb*. Palmer Lake: Filter Press, 1970.

Lloyd, William. *The Endowment and Founding of the Myron Stratton Home; or The First Decade of a Village Institution (1902–1917)*. Denver: The State Board of Charities and Corrections, 1912.

McKay, Douglas R. "Chasing the Cure at Nordrach Ranch: A History of Colorado's First Sanatorium of the Open Air." *The Colorado Magazine* 56 (Winter-Spring 1979): 179-95.

MacLaren, Thomas. "The Cragmor." *American Architect and Building News*, April 7, 1906.

———. "Sanatoria for Consumptives." *The Brickbuilder* 17 (September 1908).

Marshall, Lawrence W. "Early Denver History as Told by Contemporary Newspaper Advertisements." *The Colorado Magazine* 8 (September 1931): 161–72.

Matthiessen. F. O. *Russell Chaney (1881–1945): A Record of His Work*. New York: Oxford University Press, 1947.

Mecca (Denver) 4 (May 3,1902).

Mountain Sunshine (Colorado Springs). Vol. 1 (June 1899-May 1900); Vol. 2 (September-November 1900).

The New Cragmor (pamphlet). Colorado Springs: Cragmor Sanatorium, ca. 1936.

Ninety-Eight-Six. Colorado Springs: The Cragmor Sanatorium. Published from July 16, 1924, through February 25, 1932 (first issue called *The Cragmor News*).

The Nordrach Ranch Sanatorium and Hotel Company (pamphlet). 5th ed., Colorado Springs: Nordrach Ranch, 1905.

Ormes, Manly Dayton and Eleanor R. Ormes. *The Book of Colorado Springs*. Colorado Springs: Denton Printing Company, 1933.

Parsons, Eugene. *The Making of Colorado*. Chicago: A. Flanagan Co., 1908.

Quiett, Glenn C. *They Built the West*. New York: Appleton-Century, 1934.

Rehabilitation Center: 1928–1953 (pamphlet). Colorado Springs: Half-Way House, 1953.

Rollier, A. *La cure de Soleil*. Paris: Bailliere et Fils, 1915.

Sack, Gudrun T. "The Half-Way House."*Ent-ries* 6 (October 1956).

St. Clair, Boyd. "The Cragmor Sanatorium." *Hospital Topics and Buyer* 6 (April 1928): 262–66.

Schaefer, Samuel and Eugene Parsons. "A Brief History of the National Jewish Hospital at Denver." *The Colorado Magazine* 5 (October 1928): 191–98.

Seitz, Don C. *Joseph Pulitzer: His Life and Letters.* New York: Simon and Schuster, 1924.

The Shooks Run Inventory of Historic Sites. Colorado Springs City Planning Department, 1979.

Solly, Samuel Edwin. *An Appeal for The Cragmor Sanatorium Association* (pamphlet). Colorado Springs: Cragmor Sanatorium, May 1, 1902.

———. *Colorado Springs, Colorado, at the foot of Pike's Peak . . . together with a Collection of Medical Facts concerning Colorado Springs.* Colorado Springs: Privately printed, 1892.

———. *Facts, Medical and General, Concerning Colorado Springs, Colorado.* 2d ed., rev. Colorado Springs: Gazette Printing Company, 1895.

———. *A Handbook of Medical Climatology.* Philadelphia and New York: Lea Bros. and Company, 1897.

———. *The Health Resorts of Colorado Springs and Manitou.* Colorado Springs: Gazette Publishing Company, 188[-].

———. *Manitou, Colorado, U.S.A., Its Mineral Waters and Climate.* St. Louis: McKittrick and Company, 1875.

Solly, Samuel Edwin, Charles Fox Gardiner, and G. McClurg. *The Colorado Springs Region as a Health and Pleasure Resort: High Altitudes for Invalids.* Revised by a Committee of the El Paso County Medical Society and the Secretary of the Colorado Springs Chamber of Commerce, 1903 and 1908.

Sprague, Marshall. *The Business of Getting Well.* New York: Thomas Y. Crowell Company, 1943.

———. "Healers in Pikes Peak History." *The 1967 Denver Westerners Brand Book* 23 (1968).

———. *Newport in the Rockies: The Life and Good Times of Colorado Springs.* Denver: Sage Books, 1961.

———. *One Hundred Plus: A Centennial Story of Colorado Springs.* Colorado Springs Centennial, Inc., 1971.

———. "A Toast to Dr. Solly! (1889–1897)." *El Paso Club—A Century of Friendship.* Colorado Springs, 1976.

Stoner, Stanley. *Some Recollections of Robert Reid.* Colorado Springs: Denton Printing Co., 1934.

Stubbert, J. Edward. "Tent Life for Consumptives." *Transactions of the American Climatological Association,* 19 (1903).

The Sun Cure at Cragmor (pamphlet). Colorado Springs: Cragmor Sanatorium, ca. 1926.

Swan, Will H. "Impressions of Differences in Practice at Low and High Altitudes." *Philadelphia Medical Journal,* April 4, 1903.

Swanberg, W. A. *Pulitzer.* New York: Charles Scribner's Sons, 1967.

"Tent Cottages for Consumptives." *Charities Review* 10 (May 9, 1903).

A Trip to the Modern Woodmen of America Sanatorium at Woodmen, Colorado (pamphlet). Modern Woodmen Press, 1925.

Trudeau, Edward Livingston. *An Autobiography.* Garden City, NY: Doubleday, Page and Company, 1916.

Webb, Gerald B. "The Prescription of Literature." *The Diplomat* (Phila-
delphia), March, 1933.
———. "The Role of the Physician in Literature." *Medical Life* (1929)
(Reprinted from *Ninety-Eight-Six*).
———. *Tuberculosis*. New York: Paul B. Hoeber, 1936.
Webb, Gerald B. and Desmond S. Powell. *Henry Sewell, Physiologist
and Physician*. Baltimore: The Johns Hopkins Press, 1946.
Webb, Gerald B. and Charles T. Ryder. *Overcoming Tuberculosis: An Al-
manac of Recovery*. New York: Paul B. Hoeber, 1927.
Webb: Physician and Scholar, 1871–1948. Webb Memorial Pamphlet,
1948.
Wilson, Julius Lane. "Pikes Peak or Bust: An Historical Note on the
Search for Health in the Rockies." *Rocky Mountain Medical Journal* 64
(September 1967): 58-62.
Winning Health in the Pikes Peak Region (pamphlet). Colorado Springs
Chamber of Commerce, 1923.

UNPUBLISHED SOURCES

Cragin, F. W. Notebooks. Pioneers' Museum, Colorado Springs, Colo-
rado.
Cragin, Laurence L. Papers and Correspondence. Special Collections,
Tutt Library, Colorado College, Colorado Springs, Colorado.
Cragmor Sanatorium Company, Inc. Minutes of Executive Meetings,
Correspondence, Affidavits, Receipts, and Financial Reports Span-
ning the Years 1914–1936.
Cragmor Foundation, Inc. Minutes of Board of Directors, Record of
Proceedings, Correspondence, and Financial Reports Dated from
February 13, 1936, to May 26, 1965.
Cragmor Sanatorium Patient Ledger. Admission Records, Medical No-
tations, and Sputum/Temperature Charts, 1910–1924 (incomplete).
Forster, Alexius M. Private Papers, Miscellaneous Medical Publications,
Letters, Memoranda. Courtesy Evelyn Martin of Colorado Springs,
Colorado, and Josianne Doyle of Phoenix, Arizona.
Foster, Helen T. "The Origins of the University of Colorado at Colorado
Springs, 1952–1975." Master's thesis, University of Colorado at
Colorado Springs, 1976.
Freed, Elaine. "Thomas MacLaren Designs," undated.
Gulliford, Andrew. "Come Only if Rich: The Health-Seeker Movement
in Colorado Springs," Unpublished Paper, 1947. Special Collections,
Tutt Library, Colorado College, Colorado Springs, Colorado.
MacLaren, Thomas. Architectural Drawings, Blueprints, Maps, Colorado.
Springs and Vicinity. Western History Collection, Pikes Peak Pub-
lic Library, Colorado Springs, Colorado.

Ormes, Manly D. Papers. Special Collections, Tutt Library, Colorado College, Colorado Springs, Colorado.

Pace, J. G. Papers. Modern Woodmen of America Sanatorium, ca. 1921, Colorado Springs, Colorado.

Palmer, William J. Notebooks, Diaries, and Letters. Pioneers' Museum, Colorado Springs, Colorado.

Receiving Sheet and Receipt, Estate of Liana Forster. Pioneers' Museum, Colorado Springs, Colorado.

Solly, Samuel Edwin. Private Papers, Scrapbook, Clippings, Letters, and Notations (ca. 1887–1905).

Sprague, Marshall. "Healers in Pikes Peak History." Address, October 18, 1966.

————. Personal notes on Cragmor Sanatorium; mss. of public addresses.

Stone, Henry Chase. Papers, Diaries, Letters. Western History Collection, Pikes Peak Public Library, Colorado Springs, Colorado, and Mead Stone.

Walters, Thomas A. "Thomas MacLaren and Colorado Springs' North End" Unpublished Article, Denver.

Webb, Gerald B. Papers. Courtesy Mrs. John W. Stewart and the Webb Memorial Library, Penrose Hospital, Colorado Springs, Colorado.

INDEX

The following list is limited to those individuals mentioned in the text and footnotes who played a role in the Cragmor/Colorado Springs story.

Grateful acknowledgment is made to the following for permission to use illustrations from their collections: Pikes Peak Library, Local History Collection, Colorado Springs, pp. 6, 23, 54, 92; Tutt Library, Special Collections, Colorado College, Colorado Springs, pp. 13, 54-55, 76, 85, 101; Laura Gilpin, pp. 76, 85; Frieda Lochthowe, pp. 32, 131; Penrose Hospital, Colorado Springs, p. 59; Mead Stone, p. 92; Agnes Dwire, pp. 92, 93, 140; Gussie Templeton, p. 93; Lew Tilley and Virginia Dykstra, pp. 146-47.